Principles of
Veterinary Radiography

Principles of Veterinary Radiography

S. W. Douglas MA, MRCVS, DVR

M. E. Herrtage MA, BVSc, MRCVS, DVR

H. D. Williamson MA, BA, DCR

Department of Clinical Veterinary Medicine
University of Cambridge

FOURTH EDITION

Baillière Tindall London Philadelphia Toronto
Mexico City Sydney Tokyo Hong Kong

Baillière Tindall   33 The Avenue
W.B. Saunders   Eastbourne, East Sussex BN21 3UN, England

West Washington Square
Philadelphia, PA 19105, USA

1 Goldthorne Avenue
Toronto, Ontario M8Z 5T9, Canada

Apartado 26370—Cedro 512
Mexico 4, DF Mexico

ABP Australia Ltd, 44–50 Waterloo Road
North Ryde, NSW 2113, Australia

Ichibancho Central Building, 22–1 Ichibancho
Chiyoda-ku, Tokyo 102, Japan

10/fl, Inter-Continental Plaza, 94 Granville Road
Tsim Sha Tsui East, Kowloon, Hong Kong

First published 1963
Third edition 1980
Fourth edition 1987

Typeset, printed and bound in Great Britain by
Butler and Tanner Ltd, Frome and London

British Library Cataloguing in Publication Data
Douglas, S.W.
   Principles of veterinary radiography.—
   4th ed.
   1. Veterinary radiography
   I. Title   II. Herrtage, M.E.
   III. Williamson, H.D.
   636.089'60757   SF757.8
ISBN 0–7020–1176–2

Contents

vi   *Contents*

Since the last edition of this book was published, *Principles of Veterinary Radiography* has 'come of age' and is now in its third decade. This period has been marked by an even more rapid expansion of the use of radiography in veterinary medicine, and with the help of Michael Herrtage, who has joined the editorial team, a particularly extensive revision of the work has been undertaken.

The purpose of this book remains unchanged and is that of providing theoretical and practical guidance for students and practitioners in the safe and efficient use of radiography in veterinary practice. In the new edition, however, the authors have also endeavoured to produce a book of reference for veterinary nurses, who are now playing an increasingly important part in veterinary radiography, and for those practitioners who, having developed a particular interest in the subject, are studying for the Certificate in Veterinary Radiology of the Royal College of Veterinary Surgeons. While *Principles of Veterinary Radiography* was written primarily for use in the United Kingdom, the authors have been gratified to find that it has been welcomed and used throughout the world. The needs of this wider circle of readers have been kept in mind and it is believed that this new edition will continue to be of value to our veterinary colleagues overseas.

Those familiar with earlier editions of this work will find that the extensive revision mentioned above has involved practically every chapter of the book. Part One commences with a more detailed consideration and explanation of the theoretical physical principles which underlie the practice of radiography, and this is followed in subsequent chapters by an updating and expansion of the information on X-ray machines, accessory apparatus and processing techniques. Also in the first part of the book, the publication and implementation in the United Kingdom of new guidelines and legislation concerning the safe use of radiography has necessitated a further rewriting of the chapter on radiation protection.

In Part Two all the positions advocated for radiography of the dog and horse have been reviewed with regard to their suitability for optimum demonstration of the part concerned and the practicability and safety of the procedure necessary to undertake this. As a result of this, the majority of positions have been adapted to make greater use of the vertical X-ray beam. Chemical restraint and positioning aids are advised rather than manual restraint. Consequently, it has been necessary to redraw a very large number of the positioning diagrams in order to illustrate these changes fully. These positions have now been retitled to conform with the new anatomical terminology, which is required for scientific publications, but, to avoid too much confusion, the older, more familiar, descriptions have also been retained. The chapter concerned with the less usual species of patient contains useful information for the veterinary surgeon who may be asked to undertake the repeated radiography of laboratory animals, but the cat is now accorded a separate chapter which includes a comprehensive series of radiographs demonstrating the normal anatomy of this species. The chapter on the use of contrast media has also been extensively revised and brought up to date with regard both to the agents and to the techniques for which they are used.

This work has continued to be a product of the University of Cambridge Department of Clinical Veterinary Medicine and the authors gratefully acknowledge the help and encouragement they have received from all their colleagues. In particular they wish to thank Ruth Dennis for her practical help, advice and criticism and Andrew Sharpe, who produced a number of the photographs and has continued the contribution made by the Department's earlier photographers. Special thanks are also due to Joss Herrtage for invaluable help with the typing.

S. W. Douglas
M. E. Herrtage
H. D. Williamson

We are also indebted to the School of Radiography of the Derbyshire Royal Infirmary for technical advice and facilities and to the Equine Centre of the Animal Health Trust for the illustrations on pp. 31 and 32.

PART 1

THEORY AND EQUIPMENT

The production of a radiograph involves the use of complicated apparatus and a sequence of complex physical processes. Fortunately the controls of the X-ray machine are relatively simple and it is not necessary for the veterinary radiographer to have a detailed knowledge of the underlying radiological physics, but there are certain aspects of the subject where a basic understanding of the principles will allow the radiographer to make the best use of the equipment available. This chapter will be concerned with the physics involved in the production of X-rays within an X-ray tube and the subsequent interaction of the X-rays with matter. The succeeding chapters will deal with other aspects of X-ray machines, the properties of the X-ray beam, and the recording and visualization of the image produced.

Chapter 1

The Fundamental Physics of Radiography

THE ELECTROMAGNETIC SPECTRUM

X-rays form only one part of the spectrum of electromagnetic radiation, which includes radio waves, microwaves (radar, heating etc.), infra-red, visible light, ultraviolet light, X-rays and gamma rays (Fig. 1.1). These radiations do not require a medium

Fig. 1.1 The electromagnetic spectrum.

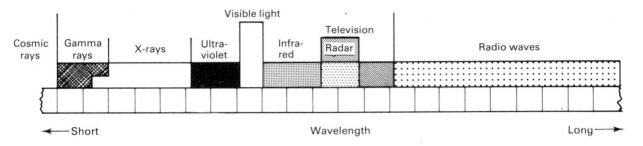

for transmission and are capable of being propagated through a vacuum. They are all transmitted by combined electric and magnetic fields and travel with the same velocity in a vacuum, i.e. 3×10^8 m/s. They travel in straight lines and when they interact with matter they can be absorbed or scattered. Electromagnetic radiation has characteristics of both transverse waves and discrete particles.

The parts of the electromagnetic spectrum are distinguished from one another by their wavelength, frequency and energy. They travel as transverse waves in which the motion of a particle is perpendicular to the direction of movement of the wave (Fig. 1.2). The distance between two particles at similar consecutive points on the waveform is the wavelength (λ). The frequency (v)

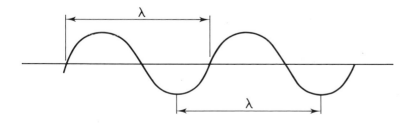

Fig. 1.2 Wave motion indicating wavelength.

of the wave is the number of cycles of the wave which pass a fixed point per second. The velocity (c) is the distance travelled forward by a point on the wave and is equal to the wavelength multiplied by the frequency:

$$c = \lambda \times v$$

where c = the velocity (3×10^8 m/s in a vacuum)
λ = the wavelength of the radiation
v = the frequency of the radiation

Since the velocity in a given medium is the same for all electromagnetic waves, it can be seen that the wavelength is inversely proportional to the frequency. Thus X-radiation, with its short wavelength, has a correspondingly high frequency.

At any point in an electromagnetic wave, there is an oscillating electric field perpendicular to the direction of the wave and an oscillating magnetic field perpendicular to both the electric field and the direction of the wave, hence the name *electromagnetic radiation*.

The wave theory gives a good account of the transmission of electromagnetic radiation, but it is often convenient to assume that a beam of electromagnetic radiation delivers its energy as a series of discrete packets of energy known as *quanta*. A quantum of electromagnetic energy is also called a *photon*. It has no mass or electric charge and consists solely of energy. The energy of a photon is determined by its frequency:

$$\varepsilon = h \times v$$

where ε = the energy of the quantum or photon
h = a constant known as Planck's constant (6.6×10^{-34} Js)
v = the frequency of the radiation

Since the frequency of a given radiation is inversely proportional to its wavelength, substitution in the above equation means that the quantum or photon energy is inversely proportional to the wavelength of the radiation, i.e. $\varepsilon \alpha \frac{1}{\lambda}$. Thus X-rays with short wavelength have photons of high energy. The high photon energy of X-rays is usually expressed in units of 1000 electron volts, or kiloelectron volts (keV), not to be confused with the kilovoltage (kV) settings on the X-ray machine.

THE PROPERTIES OF X-RAYS

The short wavelength, high frequency and high energy of X-ray photons give them properties useful in diagnostic radiology. These properties are additional to those of all the electromagnetic radiations mentioned above and can be grouped under the following headings:

1 *Fluorescence.*   X-rays cause certain substances to fluoresce, e.g. calcium tungstate or the so-called rare-earth phosphors. Fluorescence is the property possessed by certain crystalline substances of emitting characteristic radiation within the visible spectrum after absorbing electromagnetic radiation of a shorter wavelength.

2 *Photographic effect.* X-rays produce a 'latent image' on photographic film which can be made visible by processing the film.

3 *Penetration.* X-rays have the ability to penetrate substances or tissues that are opaque to visible light. They are gradually absorbed the further they pass through an object. The amount of absorption depends on the atomic number and the density of the object and on the energy of the X-rays.

4 *Excitation and ionization.* X-rays produce excitation and ionization of the atoms and molecules of the substances, including gases, through which they pass. Excitation is a process where an electron is moved to a higher energy level but still remains within the atom. Energy is required to initiate this transition and when the electron returns to its normal shell, an equivalent amount of energy is released as heat. Ionization, however, is a process in which an electron (usually an outer one) is completely removed from the atom so that the atom is left positively charged. More energy is required to initiate this process. When an electron returns to fill the space in the shell, energy is released as heat.

5 *Biological effects.* X-rays interact with living tissue and can cause biological changes, either by the direct action of excitation and ionization on important molecules in the cells or indirectly as a result of chemical changes occurring near the cells. Affected cells may be damaged or killed. The biological effects are of two types: those which damage the chromosomes or cause mutation of genes in the reproductive cells (thus affecting future generations) are known as *genetic effects*, whereas those which are evident during an individual's lifetime (e.g. radiation burns or leukaemia) are known as *somatic effects*.

THE PRODUCTION OF X-RAYS

X-rays are produced whenever charged particles are slowed down or stopped. The output of X-radiation is inversely proportional to the square of the mass of the incident particles. Electrons are used because of their small size. When fast-moving electrons are slowed down or stopped, X-rays are produced by two different processes.

In the first process, the incident electron passes close to the nucleus of an atom and its attraction to the positive electric charge on the nucleus causes it to decelerate rapidly. The electron loses energy which is emitted in the form of an X-ray photon (Fig. 1.3).

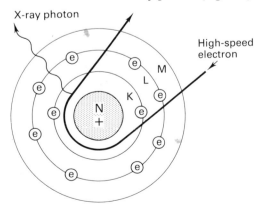

Fig. 1.3 Bremsstrahlung radiation.

The energy of the X-ray photon depends on the degree to which the electron is decelerated by its attraction to the nucleus. This process can therefore result in X-ray photons of energies from zero up to a maximum value which is equal to the total energy of the incident electron. The X-radiation produced by the deceleration of electrons is known as *Bremsstrahlung* or *braking radiation*. It gives rise to the *continuous spectrum* of X-rays, in which the intensity of the X-rays is continuous over a range of wavelengths. If intensity is plotted against photon energy for the continuous spectrum the result is shown in Fig. 1.4.

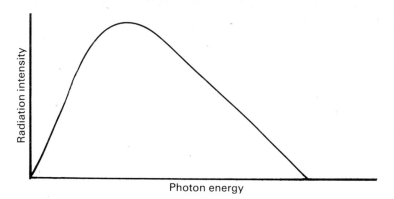

Fig. 1.4   The continuous spectrum.

The second process occurs when the incident electron collides with an electron from an inner shell of an atom and transfers sufficient energy to eject that electron from the atom. To do this, the incident electron must have energy equal to or exceeding the binding energy for that shell. An outer electron falls into the vacancy and when this transition occurs, it is accompanied by the emission of an X-ray photon of a particular energy, which is equal to the difference between the binding energies of the two shells involved in the transition. Transitions from outer orbits to the K or innermost shell result in a group of similar energies, called K peaks, and transitions to the L shell result in a group of lower energies, the L peaks. The difference in energy levels depends only on the target atom and is characteristic for that element (Fig. 1.5). The *characteristic* or *line spectrum* therefore occurs only at a

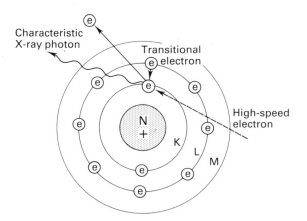

Fig. 1.5   Characteristic radiation.

few wavelengths for each element. Superimposing this characteristic spectrum on the continuous spectrum is shown in Fig. 1.6.

In practice, many of the fast-moving electrons will not produce X-rays when they interact with atoms but will give up their kinetic energy as heat. This comes from excitation or ionization of atoms involving electrons in the outer shells. In fact, in diagnostic X-ray tubes 99 per cent of the energy from fast moving electrons is converted into heat and only 1 per cent into X-ray energy.

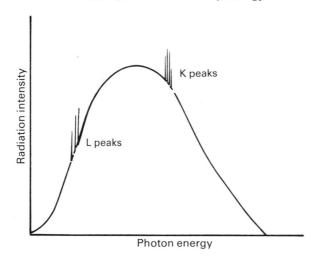

Fig. 1.6   The characteristic (line) spectrum superimposed on the continuous spectrum.

THE X-RAY TUBE

Since X-rays are produced when fast-moving electrons are slowed down or stopped, there are three basic requirements for X-ray production in a X-ray tube: (1) a source of electrons; (2) a target to stop the electrons and (3) a method of accelerating the electrons from the source to the target.

An X-ray tube consists of an evacuated glass tube into which are sealed two electrodes, the cathode (negative) and the anode (positive) (Fig. 1.7). A high vacuum exists in the tube so that there is no gas present, as this could produce electrons by ionization.

The cathode

The cathode is the electron source and the negative electrode for the high voltage placed across the tube. Electrons are produced by heating a filament, which is usually a spiral of thick tungsten wire, by passing an electric current through it from the low-tension circuit of the X-ray machine (Fig. 2.1, see page 19). This process is known as *thermionic emission*. When a metal is heated, the movement and velocity of the outer or 'free' electrons increases and a temperature can be reached where the electrons have sufficient velocity to pass through the surface of the metal and form an electron cloud around the metal. Tungsten is used because of its good mechanical properties and its ability to be heated to high temperatures for thermionic emission.

The number of electrons available to the electron cloud is directly proportional to the temperature of the filament. The num-

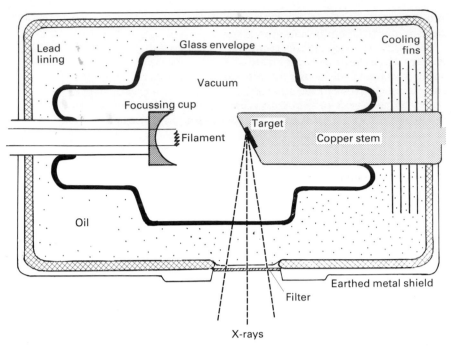

Fig. 1.7   Diagram of a fixed anode X-ray tube.

ber of electrons which pass from the cathode to the anode during an exposure represents the *tube current* and is measured in *milliamperes* (mA). Therefore, by regulating the current which heats the filament, the radiographer can control the tube current.

Since the electrons tend to repel each other, there is a tendency for the electron stream to spread out as it crosses the tube. The filament is therefore positioned in a focussing cup, usually made of nickel or molybdenum, which is maintained at the same negative potential as the heated filament. The focussing cup shapes the electrical lines of force in the tube so that the electrons are confined to a narrow stream directed towards a relatively small area of the target.

The anode

Opposite the cathode is the anode which consists of the target material embedded in a cylinder or disc, depending on whether it is a fixed or rotating anode X-ray tube. During an exposure, the anode is maintained at a high positive potential relative to the cathode. Electrons emitted from the filament are accelerated towards the anode and strike the target, which is usually made of tungsten or a tungsten–rhenium alloy. The kinetic energy of the electrons when they reach the target is proportional to the high voltage which has accelerated them across the tube. The potential difference between the anode and the cathode is measured in *kilovolts* (kV). The higher the kilovoltage, the faster the electrons are accelerated and the greater the energy of the X-rays that are produced when the electrons strike the target. However, as mentioned above, less than 1 per cent of the energy brought by the electrons to the target of a diagnostic tube is converted into X-ray energy. More than 99 per cent of the energy is converted into heat energy. Thus the construction of the anode is designed to remove heat from the target.

Tungsten or tungsten–rhenium alloy is used for the target because of its high melting point (3380°C), adequate thermal conductivity and its high atomic number (74) which increases the efficiency of X-ray production.

In a *fixed anode* X-ray tube, the tungsten target is a rectangle or disc about 1 mm thick embedded in a large cylinder of solid copper. It is set in copper because copper is a good thermal conductor and conducts the heat away from the target as rapidly as possible. The heat passes into the oil which surrounds the glass envelope and metal fins at the end of the anode stem are used to facilitate the removal of heat from the anode to the oil. Stationary anodes are used in portable and dental X-ray machines.

The *rotating anode* X-ray tube (Fig. 1.8) is able to carry a higher load than a fixed anode tube because the target area of impact for the electrons on the anode is greatly increased, so the heat produced can be spread over a much greater area. The anode consists of a disc of molybdenum with a tungsten or tungsten-rhenium alloy inset on the flange at the edge of the disc. The disc is mounted on a molybdenum rod which is rotated at high speed by an induction motor. The induction motor consists of rotor windings, which are inside the glass envelope and require no electrical supply, and the stator windings which are energized from the mains and are mounted outside the glass envelope. The induced electromagnetic force in the rotor causes it to rotate the anode at speeds of 3000 rev/min and up to 10,000 rev/min in some modern tubes. The bearings carrying the rotating shaft are lubricated with a dry lubricant and normally last the whole life of the tube.

Fig. 1.8 Diagram of a rotating anode X-ray tube.

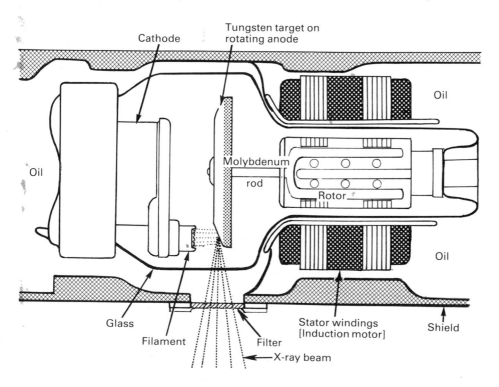

Cathode

Tungsten target on rotating anode

Oil

Oil

Molybdenum rod

Rotor

Oil

Glass

Filament

Filter

Stator windings [Induction motor]

Shield

←X-ray beam

Molybdenum is used for the rod and backing disc because of its good mechanical properties and also because it is not a particularly good conductor of heat. In this type of tube it is undesirable to conduct heat down the anode stem because this could cause a dangerous rise in temperature of the bearings and the motor. Heat is lost almost entirely by radiation from the target to the outer glass wall.

Rotating anode tubes are used in high-powered mobile and fixed X-ray machines because of the increased ability of this type of tube to dissipate heat.

The tube, with either type of anode, is surrounded by an earthed metal case to make it shock proof. This outer casing is lined with lead to prevent leakage of X-rays except in the region opposite the anode from which the X-ray beam will emerge (the *window*). The space between the case and tube is filled with oil to provide both insulation and cooling.

THE FOCAL SPOT

Ideally, the origin or focus of an X-ray beam used in diagnostic radiography should be a point source in order to get the sharpest image. However, if it is to sustain the heat produced during an exposure, it should be as large as possible. Thus a compromise has to be reached.

This is achieved by setting the target at an angle to the direction of the beam so that the area over which the electrons impinge is greater than the apparent area from which X-rays are produced when viewed along the axis of the X-ray beam. If the target is angled too steeply, the primary beam can cover only a very restricted area since the X-rays would be absorbed by the target

Fig. 1.9   Diagram of the filament-anode assembly showing: (i) coarse and fine focus; (ii) fixed anode target; (iii) actual and effective focus.

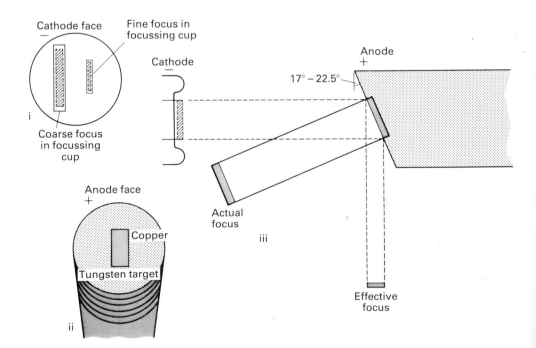

and anode. The area of the target covered by the electron beam is largely determined by the size and shape of the filament.

In a diagnostic tube, the target is usually angled to about $20°$ from the vertical (Fig. 1.9). The actual focal spot is the area on the target face receiving the bombardment by electrons and is some three times the size of the effective focal spot, which is the area projected in the direction of the X-ray beam. The effective focus is likely to be within the range $0.3–2 \, mm^2$. Some tubes provide a choice of two sizes, the smaller or *fine focus* being used when fine detail is required in the radiograph and when the output of the machine and thus heat produced can be restricted. The larger or *coarse focus* is used when it is necessary to subject the tube to a heavier current. Such X-ray tubes have two different sized filaments within the focussing cup of the cathode assembly (Fig. 1.9i).

Fixed anode tubes are limited in the load they can take because of the heat produced in the target. Rotating anode tubes enlarge the actual focal spot without affecting the size of the effective focal spot. By rotating the target, which is bevelled to an angle of about 20°, during the exposure the area subjected to electron bombardment and therefore heat production can be increased several hundred times without increasing the effective focal spot. This is why rotating anode tubes are fitted in high-powered apparatus.

THE X-RAY TUBE RATING

The subject of X-ray tube rating is complex. X-ray tube ratings dictate the maximum combinations of kV, mA, focal spot and time that can safely be used without overloading the tube. Both electrical and thermal limitations exist for a given X-ray machine.

The electrical limitations involve the maximum kV and mA. The maximum kV is determined by the design of the tube and of its shockproof housing. The quality of the electrical insulation must be sufficient to contain the high potential difference. The maximum permissible mA depends mainly on the filament design and the maximum temperature to which it is safe to heat the filament.

The thermal limitations are concerned with the tremendous amount of heat produced in the target. The dissipation of heat is affected by the physical properties of the target material, the size of the actual focal spot, the conduction of heat through the copper block in a fixed anode tube or the radiation of heat from a rotating anode tube and the rate at which heat is produced.

The production of heat is dependent on kV, mA, focal spot size and exposure time. The maximum permissible values of these for a single large exposure are usually limited by interlocks incorporated in the X-ray control console. It is wise, however, to acquaint oneself with typical exposure factors at or near the peak loading, in case the interlocking mechanism should fail. For multiple exposures taken over a short period of time, e.g. in angiocardiography, then the levels are less than those for a single exposure in order to allow for adequate cooling of the anode. The limits can be obtained from the ratings chart which is supplied for each tube by the manufacturers and takes into account both the thermal and electrical factors.

Overloading the tube can cause damage which leads to rapid deterioration and early breakdown. The tungsten target may vaporize leaving a pitted surface to the focal spot which will reduce the output of the tube. The vaporized tungsten is redeposited on the glass wall which can lead to electrical shorting. Also in simple self-rectified tubes, the heated target will emit electrons like the filament, allowing the tube current to flow in the reverse direction on the normally suppressed half cycle of the alternating current and thus wreck the delicate cathode.

The tube, therefore, must always be operated within its rating.

RECTIFICATION

High-voltage generation in X-ray equipment is closely linked with rectification which is normally achieved by the use of silicon rectifiers. In a small X-ray unit, the high-tension transformer supplies the tube with alternating current, in other words it alternately surges first in one direction and then in the other. The X-ray tube only requires current which flows in one direction – from cathode to anode. The high-tension current cannot flow from anode to cathode because the anode is 'cold' and does not have a supply of electrons to carry the current (unless the tube is overloaded). The X-ray tube itself can thus act as a rectifier suppressing the reverse cycle. This is called *self-rectification*. In apparatus in which the tube has to carry a heavier load, additional precautions have to be taken to prevent such a reversed flow of current. This is achieved by inserting two rectifiers in the circuit supplying the tube. The current will flow through the tube only during the forward half cycle. This is known as *half-wave rectification* (Fig. 1.10). The disadvantage of these systems is that only one-half of the cycle is used for the production of X-rays and short exposure times are not possible. These arrangements can only be used in portable or dental X-ray machines.

Larger apparatus is designed to make more efficient use of the current supplied to the tube. The use of four rectifiers inserted in the circuit supplying the tube enables the reverse half current to be utilized. This is known as *full-wave rectification* and allows a higher X-ray output than with a half-wave rectified circuit. However the voltage across the tube is pulsating which is a disadvantage as the intensity and quality of the X-ray beam is not as high as it would be if the voltage was constant. Also, at very short exposures (less than 0.01 s) the output will depend on the point in the cycle where the exposure starts and thus the output will vary. This type of rectification is suitable for most mobile and some fixed X-ray machines.

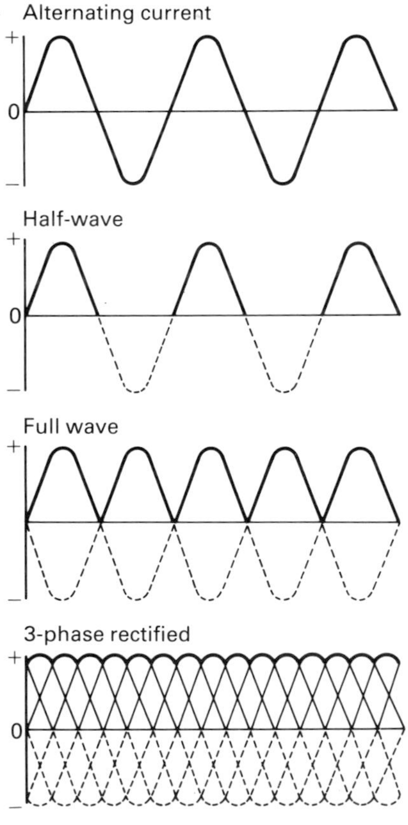

The most powerful and efficient X-ray units use either a *constant potential* generator, which is achieved by placing condensers across the output from a four rectifier circuit to maintain the voltage across the tube or a *3-phase generator* which has a 3-phase supply where there is a phase difference of one-third of a cycle between each supply (Fig. 1.10). The advantage of these arrangements is the greater output and penetrating power of the X-rays

Alternating current

Half-wave

Full wave

3-phase rectified

Fig. 1.10   Types of rectification.

for a given kV and mA, because the electrons always strike the target at the maximum kV. In addition, very short exposures times are possible since these are no longer dependent on the point in the cycle at which they begin.

Capacitor discharge generators provide a different type of power supply for producing X-rays. These units are capable of storing electrical charge in a capacitor when they are connected to an electrical supply for a short period. The generator is capable of releasing its charge rapidly to produce a short X-ray exposure. Although such units do not provide the flexibility of exposure settings available on conventional X-ray generators, they do have the advantages that they are suitable for use in remote locations and are capable of short exposure times.

It is important to appreciate that, owing to the different methods of utilizing the current, exposure factors suitable for one type of machine will bear little relationship to those necessary for another type of apparatus.

FACTORS AFFECTING THE QUALITY AND INTENSITY OF THE X-RAY BEAM

Before an X-ray tube can be used to produce X-rays it must be supplied with a suitable current of high voltage (measured in kV) and low amperage (measured in mA). It is basically these two properties of the electrical supply which control the output of the X-ray tube and the quality and intensity of the X-ray beam.

The *quality* of the beam is a measure of its penetrating power and generally the quality increases as the proportion of higher energy photons in the beam increases. Similarly, the quality increases as more of the beam has a shorter wavelength. The *intensity* is a measure of the quantity or amount of X-radiation produced. The intensity can be defined as the amount of energy flowing per second through a unit area perpendicular to the direction of the beam.

The quality and intensity of an X-ray beam are affected by various factors:

The effect of kilovoltage

The high voltage across an X-ray tube is required to accelerate the electrons towards the target in order to produce X-rays. The higher the kilovoltage employed for this purpose, the faster the electrons move, the greater the amount of energy released on impact and the higher the photon energy of the X-rays produced, i.e. the higher the quality of the beam. The maximum photon energy is proportional to the peak value of the applied voltage. In addition, the intensities of all the photon energies increase as the applied voltage is increased (Fig. 1.11). The total intensity, equivalent to the area under the curve, is approximately proportional to the applied kilovoltage squared.

The kilovoltage, therefore, affects both the quality and the intensity of the beam. The radiographer has to avoid the use of too high a kilovoltage when X-raying thin areas of tissue or all the

Fig. 1.11 Effect of increasing kV on the X-ray beam.

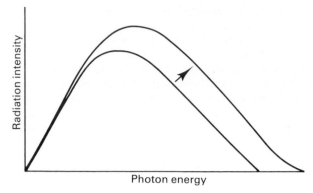

structures will be over penetrated and no differences appreciated on the film. The radiographer should select settings such that the X-rays produced are just sufficient to penetrate the densest areas of the tissues being examined. However, apparatus capable of high kilovoltage is necessary when dealing with thick or particularly dense tissue e.g. the lumbar region of large dogs or the proximal limb bones of horses.

X-rays of short wavelength and high photon energy are sometimes described as 'hard' X-rays, while those of longer wavelength and lower photon energy may be spoken of as 'soft'.

The effect of milliamperage

The amount of current which travels across an X-ray tube during an exposure depends on the number of electrons available to carry that current, which in turn varies with the current supplied to the filament and its heating effect. Altering the mA has no effect on the quality of the beam. Thus there is no change in the shape of the spectrum or in the maximum photon energy. However, the intensities of all the photon energies increase in proportion to the tube current (Fig. 1.12). The total intensity, equivalent to the area under the curve, is proportional to the average tube current.

The milliamperage, therefore, affects the intensity of the beam but has no effect on the quality of the beam. The radiographer has to adjust the current supplied to the cathode filament, usually by turning the 'milliamperage control' (see p. 22), in order to

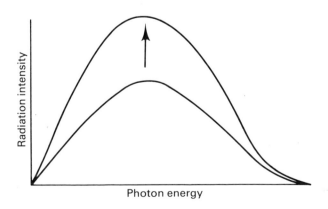

Fig. 1.12 Effect of increasing mA on the X-ray beam.

produce a sufficient quantity of X-rays to result in optimal density and detail on the radiograph.

However the quantity of X-rays produced during a given exposure also depends on the length of the exposure. Therefore the quantity of X-rays required for a given exposure is best expressed as the product of the milliamperage and time in *milliampere-seconds* (mAs).

The effect of the type of rectification

Using a constant potential or 3-phase generator instead of a pulsating waveform improves both the quality and intensity of the beam, since the average kV across the tube is increased.

The effect of the target material

Tungsten or tungsten–rhenium alloy is used for the target not only because of its high melting point and adequate thermal conductivity but also because of its high atomic number which increases the efficiency of X-ray production. The proportion of the incident energy which is converted into X-ray photons, rather than heat, is higher and thus the intensity of the X-ray beam is greater than it would be with a target containing an element with a lower atomic number.

The target material can also have a small effect on quality due to its characteristic spectrum. In the case of tungsten, the binding energy of electrons in the K shell is about 70 keV, which is within the range normally used for diagnosis.

The effect of filtration

A filter, usually a thin sheet of aluminium, is positioned across the window of the X-ray tube and will tend to absorb the lower energy photons more than the higher ones. As a result the emergent beam has a smaller proportion of low-energy photons. Its quality is therefore increased even though the total intensity is reduced (Fig. 1.13).

In diagnostic radiology, filters help reduce the dose of radiation to the superficial layers of the patient by removing the soft, low-energy rays which would otherwise be absorbed in the patient without contributing to the image on the film.

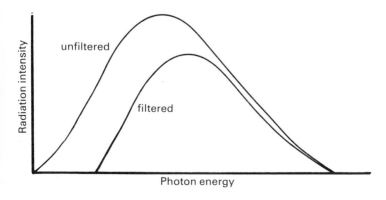

Fig. 1.13   Effect of filtration on the X-ray beam.

The effect of distance

Increasing the distance from the radiation source reduces the intensity of the beam according to the inverse square law (see p. 115) but has no effect on the quality of the beam.

From the foregoing, it can be appreciated that the radiographer has control only over the kilovoltage, milliamperage, time and distance. The method of selection of kilovoltage, milliamperage and time settings for an X-ray exposure will be discussed further in Chapter 7. It must be borne in mind that kilovoltage and milliamperage are interrelated and that, at least in the smaller types of apparatus, it is not possible to vary one without the other. In these low-powered X-ray machines, raising the kilovoltage results in reduced milliamperage.

THE INTERACTION OF X-RAYS WITH MATTER

When a beam of X-rays passes through matter its intensity is reduced. The beam is attenuated and the energy of the beam either *absorbed* by the body or *scattered*. The energy is absorbed by various processes which set electrons into motion. The kinetic energy of these electrons then produces ionization and excitation of other atoms or molecules as the electrons move through the medium. Scatter is a change in direction of a photon after inter-action with matter which may or may not be associated with a loss of energy by the photon.

There are three different processes by which X-rays used in diagnostic radiography may be absorbed or scattered when they pass through matter. They are classical scatter, photoelectric absorption and Compton scatter.

Classical scatter

Classical scatter can occur when the photons in the beam have energies which are small when compared with the binding ener-gies of electrons of the atoms or molecules in the medium. There is thus no possibility of the electron being liberated by the inter-action, but it is raised to an excited state from which it instantly returns with the subsequent re-emission of a photon of the same energy. Consequently the photon is scattered without loss of energy or change in wavelength.

This process is of little clinical significance since it never con-tributes more than 10 per cent to the overall attenuation of the incident beam and then only with radiation of long wavelength and low energy.

Photoelectric absorption

When a photon is absorbed by this process, all its energy is used up in ejecting an electron from an inner orbit of an atom (Fig. 1.14). The electron is ejected with a kinetic energy equal to the energy of the photon minus the binding energy. The displaced electron ionizes other atoms and thus converts the energy into

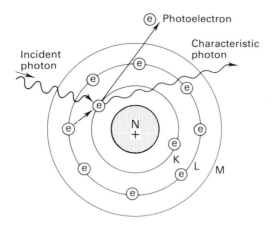

Fig. 1.14   Photoelectric absorption.

heat. The vacancy in the orbit is filled by an electron falling in from an outer orbit with the emission of characteristic radiation of the absorbing material. This radiation is usually reabsorbed within the medium.

The absorption by this process is very dependent on atomic number (Z) and is proportional to Z^3. Although it is the predominant method of absorption at low energies, its importance decreases very rapidly with increasing energy as it is inversely proportional to kV^3. It is largely the photoelectric effect that creates the *differential absorption* of the beam as it passes through a patient (see p. 39) and because of this organs and structures can be recorded on photographic film. Radiographic contrast has its origin in photoelectric absorption.

Compton scatter

This process can only occur when an incident photon has much greater energy than the binding energy of an electron in an atom of the medium. The interaction occurs with a free or loosely bound electron and only part of the photon energy is given to the electron which causes it to recoil (Fig. 1.15). The remaining energy goes

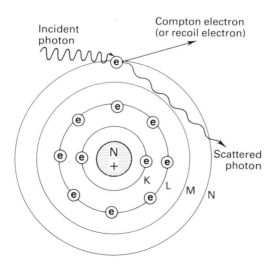

Fig. 1.15   Compton scatter.

on in the form of a scattered photon of lower energy in a different direction. The recoil electron ionizes other atoms and molecules, dissipating its energy as heat.

In this process, both scattering of the photon and absorption of energy occur. Compton absorption is independent of atomic number. It does decrease with increasing energy, though much less rapidly than for photoelectric absorption. The scattered photon can have quite a high energy and thus can be quite penetrating. It can cause a high radiation intensity outside the region irradiated by the primary beam. The importance of this process, which occurs at medium energies, is that it causes *scattered* or *secondary radiation* which tends to reduce image quality on the resultant radiograph (see p. 45).

Any X-ray apparatus, even of the simplest type, is an intricate and complicated piece of machinery, but for the purpose of this book it is sufficient to think of it as consisting of four main parts: the X-ray tube, the transformers, the tube stand and the control panel.

THE X-RAY TUBE

This has been described in the previous chapter.

THE TRANSFORMERS

Transformers are an essential part of an X-ray machine and are employed to convert the voltage of the alternating current supplied through the mains to voltages suitable for the operation of the X-ray tube.

Essentially a transformer is a device in which two coils of insulated wire are wound round an iron core. When the mains current is supplied to the first, or primary coil, a secondary current is produced in the second coil. If the number of turns of wire in the secondary coil is greater than that in the primary coil the current generated in it will be at a higher voltage than that supplied by the mains. The converse is also true, and if the number of turns in the secondary coil is less, then the voltage will be lower than that of the primary current.

Normally three different types of transformer are used (Fig. 2.1):

A high-voltage transformer is used to produce a current of a sufficiently high voltage (from 40 kV upwards) which, when

Chapter 2

The X-ray Machine

Fig. 2.1 Simplified wiring diagram of a small X-ray unit.

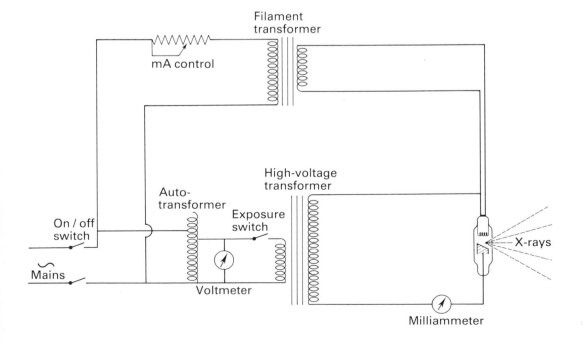

applied to the X-ray tube will permit the production of X-rays. It is a *step-up* transformer and the secondary coil contains a very large number of turns and results in the voltage being increased several hundred times. Because of the high voltages produced, these transformers have to be very carefully insulated and are normally housed in an oil bath. With small portable machines the high-tension transformer is located within the tube head and adjacent to the X-ray tube, but with more powerful machines it becomes too heavy and cumbersome to permit this. In these circumstances it is either mounted on wheels or fixed to the floor, and has to be connected to the tube by means of suitably insulated high-tension cables.

A step-down or filament transformer operates in the reverse way to the high-tension transformer and permits the supply of a suitably reduced current to heat the cathode filament.

An autotransformer is a more complicated device and consists of a single winding, part of which is used both as a primary and a secondary circuit, the two circuits being electrically connected. In effect it serves two purposes. It allows fluctuations in the mains input voltage to be corrected before the current is fed to the high-tension transformer. It also permits the voltage of that current to be varied so that the kilovoltage output of the high-tension transformer can be adjusted to that required for particular X-ray examinations.

An alternative method of generating the extremely high voltages necessary to produce diagnostic radiographs is by the use of a *capacitor-discharge generator* (see p. 28).

THE TUBE STAND

This term is used to denote the apparatus used to support the X-ray tube during the performance of radiography. It can include many different forms of suspension, and vary from small, table-top stands or larger, mobile, floor stands, to overhead ceiling mountings.

For veterinary purposes it is important that the type of stand employed should be robust, and suitable for the type of examination to be carried out. Thus, some of the lighter stands which are available are easily moved or damaged by large boisterous dogs, and a shaky stand is a common cause of movement blur on the films. Similarly, for equine work, it is essential that the stand should permit the tube head to be positioned sufficiently near to the ground for radiography of the feet.

THE CONTROL PANEL

The control panel (Fig. 2.2) contains the meters, switches and controls necessary for operating the X-ray machine and must be considered in some detail. The components of the panel will vary with different apparatus but it is likely that they will comprise some or all of the following:

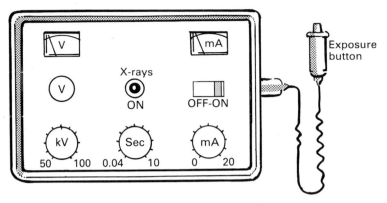

Fig. 2.2 A typical control panel of a portable X-ray machine.

The on/off switch

Provided that the machine is plugged in to a suitable live electrical socket, the closure of this switch permits the flow of current to the apparatus in anticipation of making a subsequent exposure. It is important that this control should only be left at 'on' when the machine is being used and returned to 'off' at the completion of radiography. The reason for this precaution is that, with some of the smaller and older types of apparatus, once the current is turned on the cathode filament is energized and, if left on indefinitely, may ruin the tube. Most X-ray machines are so constructed that this mishap cannot occur, but it is always wise to check that the apparatus is switched off after use and so reduce the risk of accidental exposure.

The voltmeter and voltage compensator control

An X-ray machine will not give a consistent output if there is any variation in the voltage supplied to the apparatus from the mains. The actual voltage being supplied to the machine is indicated by the voltmeter and any deviation from the normal can be corrected by adjusting the autotransformer by means of the voltage compensator control.

The kilovoltage selector

In the modern types of X-ray apparatus and in those operating on a predetermined milliamperage the kilovoltage control will be directly calibrated (usually in ascending 5 kV values) so that the desired value can be easily selected. In a number of other small machines, however, it will be found that the kilovoltage settings are indicated by a series of numbered studs and not by precise kV values. This is because the kilovoltage obtained from each setting will vary with the milliamperage being used. Such sets are normally supplied with a table giving the kilovoltage which can be expected from each stud when the machine is operated at a particular milliamperage. Examples of this arrangement are the Watson MX II (Fig. 2.6) and the A.E.I. K5 (Fig. 2.7). In yet another type of X-ray machine, the kilovoltage control is automatically linked to a certain milliampere value. This has the advantage that for low kilovoltage levels a relatively high milliamperage is available but at the other end of the scale, high kilovoltage levels are available at a low milliamperage. An example is the Japanese SMR 110/35 portable unit illustrated in Fig. 2.5. The higher stud values are: 60 kV at 25 mA, 75 kV at 20 mA, 90 kV at 15 mA and 110 kV at 10 mA.

The significance of altering the kilovoltage will be discussed further in Chapter 7, but, as already mentioned, this control affects the penetrating power of the X-ray beam produced. A range of from 45 to 75 kV is probably adequate for most small animal examinations, but slightly higher figures (up to 90 kV) can be advantageous when investigating the densest areas (e.g. the lumbar spine) of the largest dogs. Any attempt to penetrate the trunk of horses and cattle poses many additional problems but is likely to require apparatus capable of an output of at least 125–150 kV and at least 300 mA.

The milliammeter and the milliamperage selector

The milliammeter records the current passing through the tube but will only record during the actual X-ray exposure. The actual selection of the desired current is achieved by varying the current to the cathode filament but the method of doing this varies with different apparatus. In some of the smaller portable machines it is necessary to adjust the appropriate knob while making a trial exposure until the milliammeter shows the desired reading. In other apparatus the milliamperage is linked with the kilovoltage and one dial selects both, while in the majority of medium and large X-ray sets various milliamperage levels can be preselected by adjusting the control.

It will be found that the small and medium-sized X-ray apparatus cannot be set to operate at maximum milliamperage and maximum kilovoltage simultaneously.

The significance of the milliamperage is that it affects the quantity of X-rays produced and a level has to be selected which is sufficient to produce an easily recognizable image on the X-ray film without obliterating that image by over-exposure. However, the amount of radiation is also controlled by the length of the exposure and is best expressed in milliampere-seconds (i.e. the milliamperage multiplied by the time in seconds).

The timer and exposure button

The exposure button should be attached to the control panel by a length of cable so that the person making the exposure may position himself at a safe distance from the primary beam (at least two metres from the tube housing and the animal being examined).

It is necessary that the cathode filament should be activated and heated to produce electrons for a brief period before the exposure is actually made. For this reason, the exposure device in many modern units consists of a two-stage button—depression of the first half activates the filament and the rotating anode, if present, and, after a short pause, complete depression closes the circuit and makes the radiographic exposure. (As already mentioned, in some of the smaller sets the cathode filament is heated as soon as the machine is switched on.)

The adjustable timer may be located on the control panel or it may be at the end of the cable and incorporate the exposure button. There are three main types:

The clockwork timer. This timer (Fig 2.3a) is a clockwork run-back device in which the knob in the centre of the dial is turned or 'wound up' to the time required. When the exposure button is pressed the knob returns to zero and closes the circuit for the appropriate period.

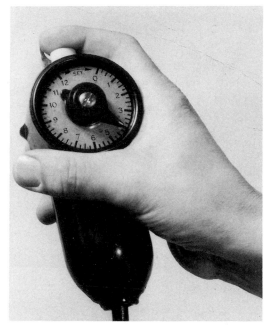

Fig. 2.3a A clockwork timer.

Such timers are usually calibrated from 0.1 or 0.125 seconds to 5 or 10 seconds. Clockwork timing devices suffer from mechanical inertia and are not completely accurate at the lowest exposure times.

Clockwork timers are the simplest and cheapest type and are usually only supplied for use with some portable machines. These timers are widely used in veterinary work but have the disadvantage that they are not very suitable for chest or other work requiring particularly brief and accurate exposures.

The synchronous timer. This timer is found in many of the larger and older machines and operates on a more intricate mechanism incorporating a synchronous electric motor. It is more accurate than a clockwork timer and permits the use of exposure times down to 0.1 seconds.

The electronic timer. This form of timer is provided with most modern sets and permits the use of very brief (0.02 seconds or less) accurately timed exposures. It is also silent in use and does not need to be reset if making repeat exposures. To operate, a dial on the control panel is adjusted to the time required and the exposure is made by pressing a button at the end of the usual long cable (Fig. 2.3b).

Since time and milliamperage have to be considered together, the advantage of being able to make very brief exposures is only of the greatest value when the apparatus is also capable of sufficient milliamperage to permit an output of the required mA-s.

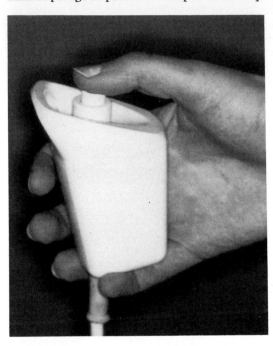

Fig. 2.3b   Two stage switch for an electronic timer.

Warning light

As a safety precaution, most control panels incorporate a warning light which is illuminated when an exposure is made and X-rays are being emitted. A further precaution, usually fitted to large installations, is for this to be linked to a second warning light located at the entrance of the X-ray room.

Fluoroscopy control

Some X-ray machines are fitted with a switch (often combined with the on/off switch) which permits the apparatus to be used either for conventional radiography or for fluoroscopy. When switched to fluoroscopy the timer is by-passed and the machine is operated for prolonged periods by depressing the exposure button (or by substituting a foot switch).

The purpose of fluoroscopy is the immediate visualization of the radiographic image by allowing the X-ray beam to impinge on a suitable fluorescent screen. This technique has been adapted and incorporated in modern image intensification apparatus (see p. 33) but here it is sufficient to state that the use of ordinary X-ray apparatus for fluoroscopic examinations involves a very serious risk of irradiation of those taking part and produces inferior radiographic demonstration of lesions, and should never be permitted.

Those portions of the control panel intended to be used for fluoroscopic purposes are frequently indicated by a symbol consisting of an 'eye', while those to be employed for ordinary radiography are marked with the outline of a simple cone (Fig. 2.4).

TYPES OF X-RAY APPARATUS

Practically all X-ray equipment used in veterinary radiography was designed and constructed for human use and suffers from various disadvantages when used for veterinary purposes. While there is a very wide variety of machines of different size, power and manufacture, they may be divided into three main groups.

Portable X-ray apparatus

Apparatus of this type is termed portable because it can easily be taken to pieces and the component parts transported by car.

In such machines (Figs 2.5–8) the transformers are of small size and low weight and are located within the tube head immediately adjacent to the X-ray tube. The tube head itself is supported on a tube stand which may comprise either a small table-top model or a considerably more substantial floor stand mounted on wheels. The apparatus also has a small control panel which is attached

Fig. 2.4   International symbols found on modern X-ray apparatus.

Off

On

Fluoroscopy

Radiography

Fig. 2.5   The Japanese-made SMR 110/35 Portable Unit mounted on an M1 stand.

Fig. 2.6   Watson M.X.II Portable Unit.

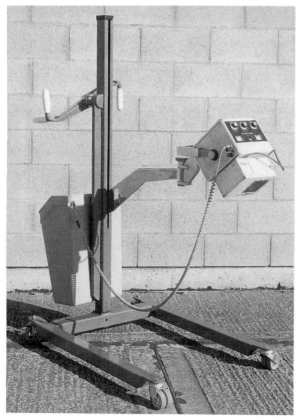

Fig. 2.5

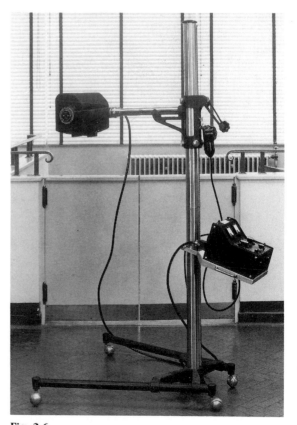

Fig. 2.6

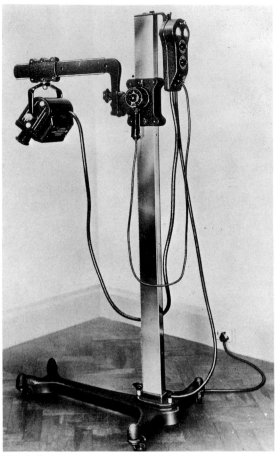

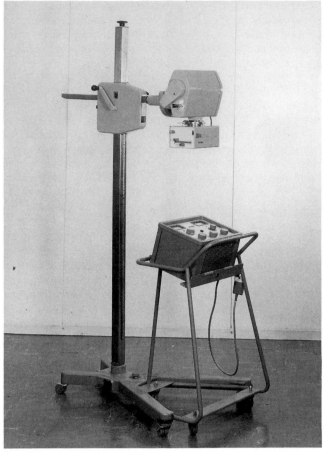

Fig. 2.7

Fig. 2.8

Fig. 2.7   The A.E.I. K5 Unit mounted on the mobile tube stand ST. 15.

Fig. 2.8   Philips Practix 20 mA Portable Unit.

to the tube stand or the tube head or supported on a separate stand.

Portable machines are the type of X-ray apparatus most widely used in general veterinary practice. They possess a number of advantages for such use:

1   They cost less than other types of machine.
2   They are strongly constructed and need little maintenance.
3   They can be operated from any 13- or 15-A electrical point.
4   They can be easily transported for use on farms or other premises.
5   They are light and easily manœuvred and therefore suitable for radiographing, for example, the legs of restless horses.

The main disadvantage of such machines is their low electrical output which limits the radiographic examinations which can be undertaken. The precise ratings vary with different makes of machine but the maximum output is likely to be from 70 to 110 kV and from 15 to 35 mA.

Range of use

The extent to which portable X-ray apparatus is suitable for general veterinary radiography depends on the radiographic technique and skill of the operator and on the capabilities of the particular machine.

The principal limiting factor is the low milliamperage which necessitates longer exposure times and thus predisposes to blurring due to movement. This problem can partly be overcome by the use of fast screens and/or films, and by anaesthetization of the patient. Given such aids, the extent of the examinations which can be satisfactorily carried out with these units will also depend on the type of animal being radiographed.

Large animals. Such machines are particularly suitable for radiography of the feet of horses but of limited use for any examination above the carpus or tarsus.

Small animals. Portable apparatus should be satisfactory for the radiographic examination of the entire skeletal system of the dog and cat (with the possible exception of the vertebral column of particularly large dogs).

There are, however, limitations on the usefulness of these smaller machines for radiography of the abdomen and chest in these species.

Provided that, where necessary, examination of the abdomen is aided by suitable techniques (compression of the abdomen to thin the part and obviate movement, the use of contrast media, etc.), it should be possible to obtain satisfactory films of the abdomen of all but the largest dogs.

To obtain good chest radiographs and to minimize the effect of respiratory movement (particularly in clinical cases showing tachypnoea) it is necessary to use exposure times of from 0.02 to 0.04 seconds. This is seldom practicable with portable apparatus because the usual clockwork timers will not permit exposures shorter than about 0.1 second. Even if suitable timers are available, the low milliamperage of these machines will limit the use of such brief exposure times to radiography of the chest of cats or small dogs. Nevertheless, in some circumstances (where respirations are slow or can be slowed, or where demonstration of gross rather than fine detail is required), such machines may be used for radiography of the chest of the medium or larger sized dog (particularly for lateral rather than dorsoventral projections).

Dental X-ray apparatus

Apparatus manufactured for dental use is sometimes advocated for veterinary use because of its low price. Such machines are of low output (in the region of 10 mA and 70 kV) and are designed to cover only a small area of the patient. The precise use which could be made of such machines would depend in part on the skill of the operator, but they are likely to be restricted to the examination of cats and the smallest dogs.

Mobile X-ray apparatus

In machines of this type (Figs 2.9–12) the transformers are larger to permit higher output and because of their increased weight are

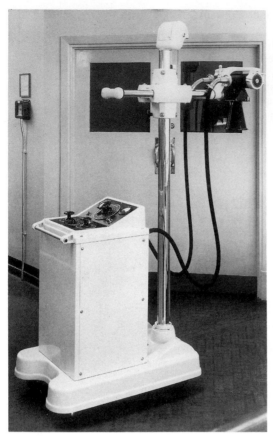

Fig. 2.9

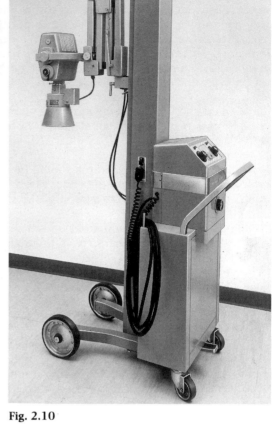

Fig. 2.10

Fig. 2.9   Watson Mobilix Ward Unit.

Fig. 2.10   General Electric Mobile *90* II.

no longer located in the tube head but are mounted on wheels and form the base of the apparatus. These sets cannot be taken apart and the tube stand and control panel are built into the apparatus. These machines can be moved over level surfaces and, in most instances, operated from 13- or 15-A sockets. However, they are somewhat cumbersome and could not be moved rapidly when dealing with a restive horse, or be transported by car.

There is considerable variation in the range of output of these units. The cheapest sets may not be capable of higher output than the portable machines. The majority produce slightly higher kilovoltage and two or three times as much milliamperage (i.e. 90 kV and 40–60 mA). The more costly units permit the use of particularly high exposure factors (a maximum of 125 kV and 300 mA) but will probably require the provision of 30-A sockets.

Capacitor discharge units are a specialized group of mobile X-ray machines which have a radiographic output comparable with the larger machines just mentioned, but which can be operated from 13-A sockets or from rechargeable batteries. The functioning of such machines is based on the fact that a capacitor is essentially a reservoir for electricity which can be charged relatively slowly to a given potential via a low-power circuit taken from the avail-

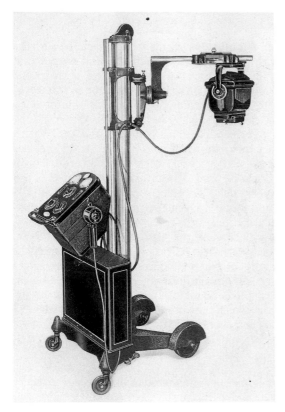

Fig. 2.11

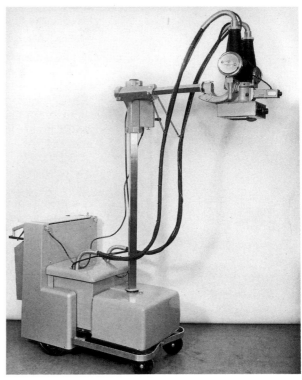

Fig. 2.12

able input voltage. Once the charge has built up to the desired kilovoltage it can be switched to the X-ray tube where it discharges in a fraction of a second. Once an exposure has been made, a short pause is necessary for recharging before the machine can be used again.

Capacitor discharge units have considerable potential for veterinary use but, like the more conventional higher powered mobile machines, are expensive and their purchase could only be justified when the number of radiographic examinations undertaken is unusually high.

Fig. 2.11   A.E.I. M.R.4 Mobile Unit.

Fig. 2.12   Dean D. 38 Mobile Unit.

Range of use

Large animals. The difficulty of manœuvring these heavier machines quickly and the fact that in many instances the tube cannot be positioned at near ground level (unless the support arm is modified) will limit its usefulness for equine work. Provided that the patient can be cast or otherwise effectively immobilized, the greater output of most of these sets will enable examination of the upper limbs, head and neck to be undertaken.

Small animals. These machines are very suitable for dog and cat work and the increased output of the medium and higher powered units would enable practically all radiographic examinations to be attempted.

Fixed X-ray apparatus

The machines which fall into this group are characterized by the fact that they require transformers of such size and output that they have to be built into the room and provided with special electrical connections to the mains. The X-ray tube is connected to the transformer by high-tension cables and is mounted on some form of gantry which allows only limited movement. Such machines are likely to be capable of an output of at least 300 mA and 120 kV and in some instances much higher (1000 mA and 200 kV). The expense of such apparatus normally restricts its use to the teaching schools and research institutes but in a few instances practitioners have installed second-hand machines obtained from a hospital at a nominal price (see note on 'second-hand apparatus' on p. 122).

The considerably increased output of such sets could be of very great advantage for veterinary purposes. However it must be appreciated that many of these machines are constructed for specific human investigations and are not necessarily suitable for general veterinary purposes. In addition, all will require large and suitably constructed rooms if they are to be used satisfactorily and safely. Other advantages and disadvantages of these machines are best considered in relation to the circumstances under which they are used.

Large animals. The higher kilovoltage and milliamperage provided by these machines should facilitate radiography of the trunk and spine of cattle and horses. However, the greatly increased amount of 'scattered radiation' (see p. 45) which is produced when higher kilovoltages are employed to penetrate greatly increased thicknesses of tissue can obliterate all detail in the radiograph. Furthermore, there will be obvious difficulties and dangers in approximating large animals and cumbersome and expensive apparatus which cannot be easily moved.

Apparatus designed specifically to overcome these problems associated with large animal radiography has been installed at certain veterinary establishments and is illustrated in Figs 2.13 and 2.14. The most important features of such apparatus are:

1   Transformers capable of an output of at least 150 kV and 500 mA (some machines go up to 200 kV and 1000 mA).
2   Ceiling mounting of the supports for the tube and film cassette so that they may be manœuvred around a horse and easily swung out of the way if the animal becomes restive.
3   Some means of accurate alignment of the X-ray tube with high ratio grids and film cassette (see Fig. 2.14) in order to minimize the effects of scattered radiation.

Small animals. Apparatus of this type is very suitable for all small animal radiographic examinations and may incorporate facilities for additional techniques such as rapid film changing, image intensification or tomography.

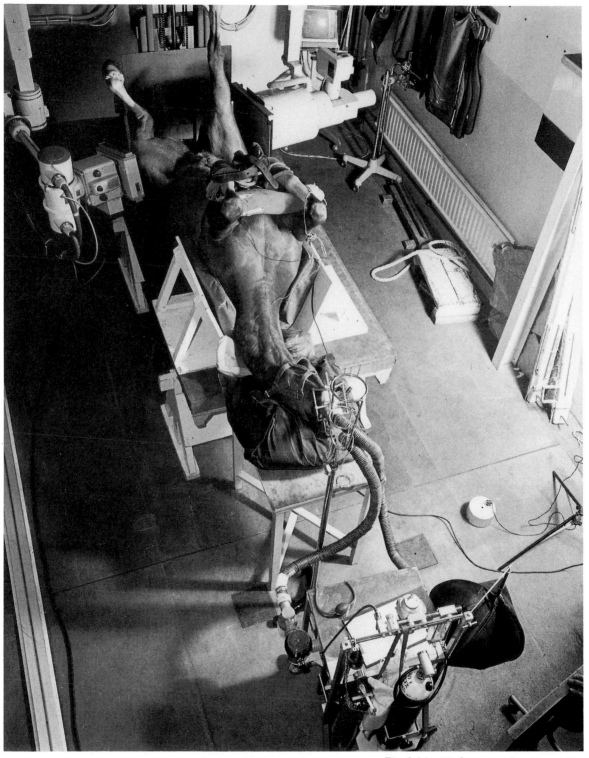

Fig. 2.13   High-powered radiographic equipment designed specifically for equine examinations.

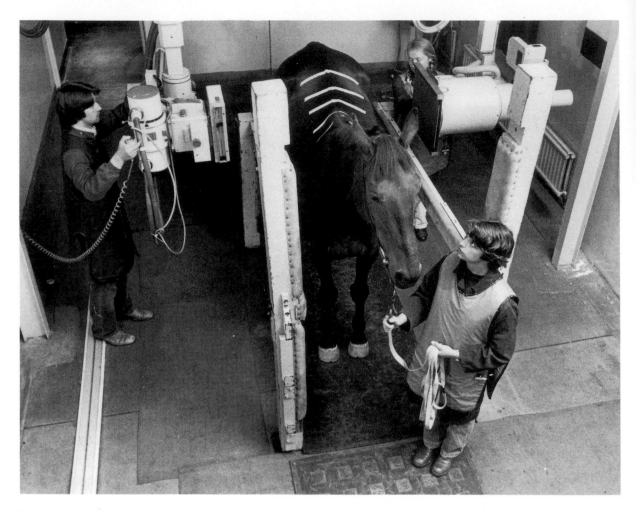

Fig. 2.14   A close-up view of the apparatus shown in Fig. 2.13. Note that the X-ray tube and cassette holder are interlocked to permit precise alignment when radiographing thick areas of tissue.

SPECIALIZED X-RAY APPARATUS

The three types of X-ray apparatus just described are intended for the production of routine radiographs and, within the limitations mentioned, are equally suitable for the investigation of veterinary and human patients. In the human field, however, some machines have been adapted for particular specialized examinations of people (e.g. apparatus designed solely for radiography of the human skull) and are unsuitable for use with animals. Some of these specialized techniques which require modified apparatus have been employed for veterinary purposes and the general principles of the two most commonly used will be described.

Fluoroscopy

The essential feature of fluoroscopy is the use of a screen containing crystals (usually zinc cadmium sulphide or caesium iodide) which fluoresce when exposed to X-rays. This screen is substituted for conventional X-ray film and is placed in the path of the diagnostic beam after it has been passed through the part of the patient under investigation. Since the intensity of the light emitted by each part of the screen is exactly proportional to the intensity of X-rays incident upon that part of the screen, the visible light pattern corresponds exactly with the X-ray pattern. The fluorescent screen thus enables the radiologist to 'see' the X-ray picture, but as a positive image (i.e. the black and white areas of a normal radiograph will be reversed).

As already mentioned, a number of older X-ray machines were fitted with fluoroscopy switches and these have been employed, in conjunction with hand-held fluorescent screens, for veterinary purposes in order to save the time and expense of exposing and developing X-ray film. Such practice must be wholeheartedly condemned, not only because the diagnostic detail which can be appreciated on a fluoroscopic screen is far less than that visible in an average radiograph, but more particularly because the amount of radiation likely to be received by all those taking part in the procedure is several hundred times that incurred in conventional radiography.

Modern fluoroscopic apparatus has been designed to minimize the above problems and is used in conjunction with an *image intensifier* which increases the brilliance of the fluoroscopic image and simultaneously enhances radiological detail and reduces the amount of radiation necessary to produce a diagnostic image.

The essential parts of an image intensifier are shown diagrammatically in Fig. 2.15. The X-ray beam is directed on to a fluorescent screen (a) which is in very close contact with a second screen composed of photoelectron-emitting material – the *photocathode* (b). These electrons are accelerated across the evacuated tube by the voltage (about 25 kV) applied between the cathode and the fluorescent viewing screen or anode (d). Absorption of the increased energy electrons in this screen produces an image which is much brighter than would be seen on the initial screen (a).

The output screen (d) is covered on the side nearest to the photocathode by a thin layer of aluminium, which permits passage of the electrons, but prevents any light travelling in the reverse

Fig. 2.15

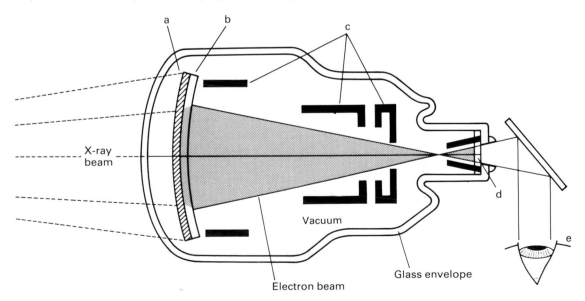

direction and reaching the photocathode. If this happened, further electrons would be liberated and, because they were not related to the pattern of the image, they would blur the detail visible in (d).

The electron lens (c) preserves the pattern of the beam of electrons but also reduces its size. The diameter of the final image is about one-fifth of that formed on the first screen (a) but its brightness is consequently increased some 25 times. This brilliance is further enhanced by the accelerating voltage and the final image will be many hundred times brighter than that received on the fluorescent screen (a). This means that the exposure factors which would normally be employed for diagnostic radiography can be considerably reduced for such examinations, thus reducing the radiation hazard involved.

One of the limitations involved in the use of an image intensifier is the small area of the patient which can be covered at any one time.

The radiographic image can be viewed directly through an eyepiece (e) but the attachment of a television camera and viewer enables the radiologist to position himself further from the X-ray beam and to share the examination with other colleagues. The addition of a video recorder or of a cine camera provides an additional facility and permits storage and retrieval of the radiographic findings (Fig. 2.16).

Image intensification apparatus used for fluoroscopic examinations should incorporate the following safety precautions:

1   The X-ray tube and screen should be on a common mounting and aligned on a common axis. Under no circumstances should the useful beam overlap the full screen area.
2   The primary beam should be restricted by an adjustable lead-shuttered diaphragm of the rectangular type and this should be mounted in a protective enclosure to prevent lateral escape of radiation.
3   The fluoroscopic stand must be provided with adequate protective arrangements of lead–rubber or lead–plywood of a lead equivalent of not less than 0.5 mm to protect the operators and staff against scattered radiation.

Tomography

Tomography is a special radiographic technique in which movement of the X-ray tube during an exposure is employed to blur the images of those parts of the patient which overlie and obscure an area of interest at a selected depth within the patient's body.

In the simplest procedure (linear tomography) the tube head and the film carrier are moved in opposite directions to each other during the radiographic exposure (Fig. 2.17).

The X-ray tube and film carrier are linked by a telescopic bar which is pivoted at its midpoint. The pivot is the crucial part of the apparatus. It must be firmly constructed and yet adjustable, so that the axis of the pivot can be arranged to correspond with the exact depth or 'slice' of the patient which it is intended to demonstrate.

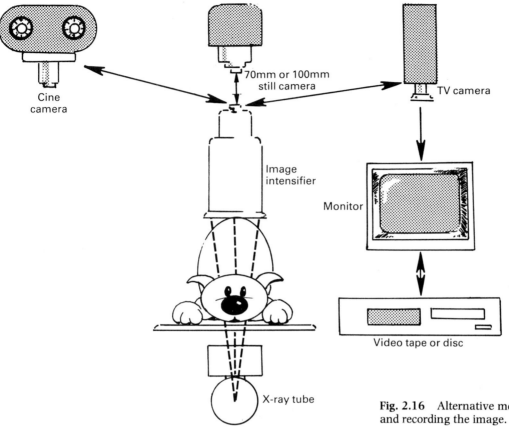

Cine
camera

70mm or 100mm
still camera

TV camera

Image
intensifier

Monitor

X-ray tube

Video tape or disc

Fig. 2.16 Alternative methods of viewing
and recording the image.

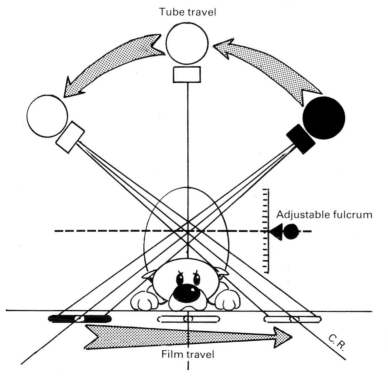

Tube travel

Adjustable fulcrum

C.R.

Film travel

Fig. 2.17 The essential features of
tomographic equipment.

Fig. 2.18 explains the effect of the technique on the radiograph. Those parts of the patient located at the level of the pivot will be reproduced consistently at P on the film. The shadowgraphs A^1 and B^1 cast by points A and B will however move from one end of the film to the other during the radiographic exposure. While this will result in an increase of diffuse density on the radiograph, the unwanted and confusing outlines of these areas will no longer be superimposed on the point of interest.

As already mentioned, only the simplest form of tomography has been described. In a slightly more intricate form of linear tomography the movements of the tube head and the film cassette describe arcs of a circle and so prevent the length of the primary beam altering during the procedure. Other tomographic systems which employ circular, elliptical or hypocycloidal motions are also available, but are unlikely to be used for veterinary purposes.

Fig. 2.18   The principle of linear tomography.

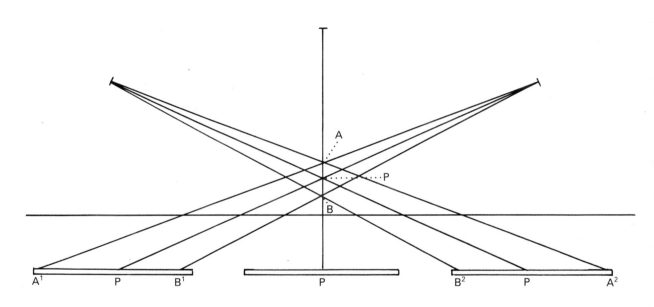

The purpose of the X-ray tubes and apparatus described in the previous two chapters is to provide a suitably controlled beam of X-rays which can be employed to demonstrate the internal structure of a patient.

Within the X-ray tube a rapidly moving stream of electrons is caused to strike a target (the anode), where part of the kinetic energy is converted into X-rays. As each electron collides with the target some of its energy is liberated as an *X-ray photon*. The X-ray beam is an aggregation of the photons resulting from millions of such collisions. The X-ray photons produced at the anode of the X-ray tube are emitted in all directions but are confined by the lead shielding surrounding the tube and only emerge, in the form of a beam, through an aperture in the shielding which is known as the *window*. The properties of this beam (sometimes described as the *primary* or *useful beam*) are considered in this chapter, particularly as it emerges from the tube head, passes through the patient, and falls on the recording medium.

THE COMPOSITION OF THE BEAM

As mentioned in Chapter 1 all X-ray beams are of mixed composition, i.e. they consist of X-rays of a range of wavelengths. Raising the kilovoltage supplied to the tube increases the proportion of short wavelength X-rays and improves the penetrating power of the beam.

Because the beam is mixed it will also contain X-rays of such long wavelength that they are incapable of penetrating any appreciable amount of tissue. Such rays do not contribute to the production of the radiographic image but do increase the amount of potentially harmful radiation received by the patient. For this reason modern apparatus incorporates additional filtration (see p. 15) provided by an aluminium filter in the tube window which prevents the passage of these useless rays.

THE COLLIMATION OF THE BEAM

The beam which emerges from the aperture of the X-ray tube is a diverging one capable of extending to a considerable width. Most X-ray machines incorporate some means of collimating or restricting this divergence to the minimum necessary to cover the area under examination. The purpose of this is three-fold:

1 To prevent unnecessary irradiation of the patient or, in veterinary radiography, of any persons involved in restraining the patient.
2 To reduce scattered radiation.
3 To minimize geometrical distortion.

In many of the simpler and older machines the restriction of the beam is accomplished by sliding an appropriate lead plate or cone (Fig. 3.1a) over the aperture of the tube immediately prior

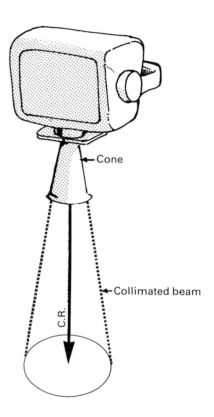

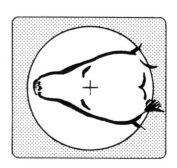

Fig. 3.1a

Chapter 3

The X-ray Beam

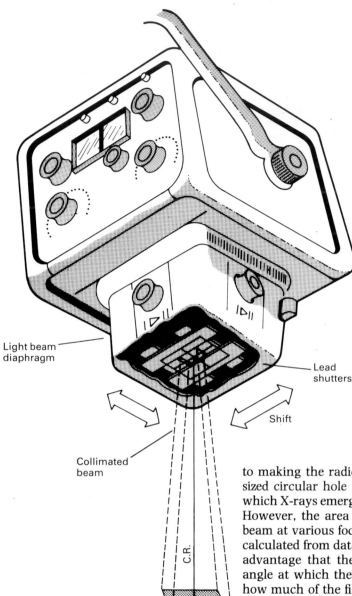

Light beam
diaphragm

Lead
shutters

Shift

Collimated
beam

C.R.

to making the radiographic exposure. Each plate has a different sized circular hole which alters the size of the window through which X-rays emerge and so controls the size of the primary beam. However, the area of the cassette which will be covered by the beam at various focal–film distances is not obvious and has to be calculated from data supplied with the apparatus. Cones have the advantage that their shape provides a visual indication of the angle at which the beam will spread and it is easier to estimate how much of the film will be exposed. Owing to the use of cones for the purpose, collimation of the beam is sometimes described as 'coning down' instead.

A more satisfactory method of restricting the beam is by means of adjustable lead shutters which are permanently attached to the tube aperture. Where, as is now usual, such devices also incorporate a source of light to visualize the extent of the primary beam, it is possible to adjust and position the beam very accurately. This addition is known as a *light beam diaphragm* (Fig. 3.1b) but it may be imperceptible in bright sunlight and is most effective when used in a semi-darkened room.

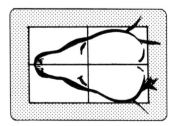

Fig. 3.1b

PENETRATION AND ABSORPTION OF THE BEAM

X-rays, because of their higher energies, have the property of penetrating matter which is opaque to visible light. This does not mean that all substances are equally radiotranslucent; if this were so, radiography would be impossible.

An average beam from a small diagnostic unit generated at 60 kV will penetrate a millimetre-thick sheet of aluminium but will be absorbed by the same thickness of lead. The radio-opacity of any substance depends upon the 'hardness' or penetrating ability of the incident beam, and also upon the *atomic number, density* and *thickness* of the material being irradiated.

The selection of control settings to obtain an X-ray beam of optimum penetrating power for any particular examination will be considered in Chapter 7.

Differential absorption

The subject of penetration and absorption is complex, and to simplify this the following example is given in which three similar theoretical rays are selected from a beam generated at 65 kV and used to radiograph a dog's thorax of 20 cm thickness (Fig. 3.2).

Ray A does not penetrate the chest at all, so that it is only slightly attenuated; in other words, only a few photons will be absorbed by air and the maximum number will pass through to the photograpic emulsion causing maximum exposure of that area of the film.

Ray B passes through the body wall which will absorb most of the long wavelength photons, but the aerated tissue of the lung is nearly as radiotranslucent as air, so the ray will be only partly attenuated and the film will receive a medium exposure.

Ray C passes through the body wall, vertebrae, mediastinum and heart. Most of the photons will be absorbed. There will be a certain amount of *scattered* radiation which will also be absorbed. Only a few photons of the highest energy will pass through to expose the film, and when the processed radiograph is examined, the area overlaid by the heart will be a relatively transparent area, in contrast to the lung shadows.

The photoelectric effect predominates up to about 60 kV but above this the Compton effect increases (see p. 16). Low kilovoltages therefore produce a high contrast between bone and soft tissue but at higher voltages contrast is reduced due to the Compton effect and the fact that more scattered radiation reaches the film.

Factors affecting radio-opacity of matter

Atomic number. This refers to the number of positive charges contained in the nucleus of the atom and equals the sum of the electrons. Each element has a specific atomic number. The substances which interest the radiographer are given in Table 3.1.

Atoms will only absorb photons of radiation of a certain energy. If the energy of the photon is greater than this, it cannot be captured by the atom. But atoms of different elements have differ-

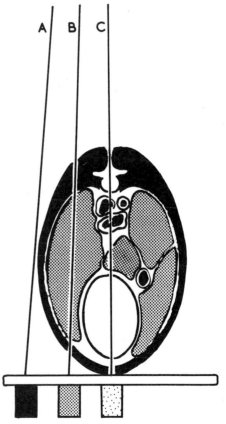

Fig. 3.2

Table 3.1   Atomic numbers.

	Element	Atomic number	
Soft tissue	Hydrogen	1	Average
	Carbon	6	of soft tissue = 6
	Nitrogen	7	
	Oxygen	8	
Bone	Calcium	20	Average of bone = 14
Photographic emulsion	Bromine	35	
	Silver	47	
Contrast media	Iodine	53	
	Barium	56	
Apparatus Tube target	Tungsten	74	
Shielding	Lead	82	

ent energy potentials, and a photon of radiation which would pass without attenuation through the atomic framework of carbon (6) would be absorbed by the more complex atomic structure of silver (47). Photographic emulsion is composed of silver halides and this is why we get the *photographic effect*. By noting the atomic number of different elements we can predict how they will absorb the X-ray beam. Bone (14) will absorb photons which pass through the atoms of soft tissue (6). The high atomic number of materials used for contrast media make it obvious why they are radio-opaque, and the use of lead for shielding against radiation is apparent because of its high atomic number.

When employing exposure factors in the lower kilovoltage range (40–60) the attenuation of an X-ray beam by substances is roughly proportional to the third power of its atomic number (see photoelectric absorption p. 16). Thus bone (14) is roughly twelve times as effective in absorbing X-rays as soft tissue (6). At higher kilovoltages, the attenuating properties of tissues have a more direct relationship to their atomic numbers.

Density. Absorption also depends upon the density of molecules of matter. This, of course, differs in solids, liquids and gases.

Air, water and soft tissue have approximately the same atomic number, but the specific gravity of air is only 0.0013, whereas water and soft tissue are 1. This fact makes air a valuable contrast medium.

Thickness. If a comparatively radiotranslucent material is thick enough, it will cause a high percentage of an X-ray beam to be absorbed.

If a beam is attenuated by 50 per cent after passing through the first centimetre of a substance, the second centimetre will reduce the beam to 25 per cent, and so on. When very thick areas of soft tissue are to be radiographed, on large animals, this factor becomes important.

THE MANIFESTATION OF THE X-RAY BEAM

Human senses cannot perceive an X-ray beam and it can be utilized only because it affects the emulsion of photographic film and produces fluorescence in certain crystals.

The photographic effect

X-rays affect photographic emulsion in almost the same way as do the photons of visible light. The emulsion consists of silver halide grains suspended in gelatin. When an X-ray or light photon hits a grain of silver halide a complex interchange of electrons takes place which liberates the halide atoms and leaves metallic silver. The effect is still invisible and is referred to as the *latent image*. The film must be placed in a developer to complete the chemical reduction of the silver halide before the image is visible.

The latent image formed by light photons is on the surface of the emulsion, but because X-ray photons can penetrate and expose silver halide grains at any depth, X-ray film emulsion is thicker than on ordinary photographic film and coated on both sides of the base. Only a small percentage of X-rays passing through a film are absorbed, so it is usual to employ *intensifying screens* which utilize the fluorescent effect of X-rays to speed up exposure of the film.

The fluorescent effect

Certain crystals, such as zinc sulphide, calcium tungstate, barium lead sulphide and the rare-earth group of compounds fluoresce when exposed to an X-ray beam. The primary X-ray photons are absorbed, and the characteristic radiation emission which results from the interchange of electrons is of the wavelength of visible light, either green or blue.

The fluorescent effect is used in diagnostic radiography in two main ways:

1 *Intensifying screens.* Calcium tungstate crystals which fluoresce blue and the rare-earth compounds, some of which fluoresce green, are coated on cards and 'sandwich' the film in a light-tight film holder, called a *cassette.* Thus light is used as well as the X-ray beam to affect the film emulsion.
2 *Direct fluoroscopy or screening.* The screens employed for fluoroscopy use zinc sulphide which fluoresces green, the colour to which the eye is most sensitive. It is used in a darkened room to visualize the structures of the patient and to observe their movements.

The biological effect of X-rays

The effect of the absorption upon the cells of the body is complicated and still not fully understood. The ionization of the atoms and the consequent disturbance to the chemistry of the cell can be harmful or even lethal after a sufficiently large dose of X-rays has been received. This damage may be caused by a single large dose or by small repeated amounts which have a cumulative effect.

THE GEOMETRY OF THE X-RAY BEAM

Since the X-ray photons that make up the primary beam travel in straight lines many of the properties of the beam can be explained and demonstrated on geometrical principles.

The intensity of the beam

The beam obeys the inverse square law i.e. for a given exposure the amount of radiation falling on a particular area (e.g. the radiographic film) will vary inversely as the square of the distance of that area from the source of irradiation (the *focal spot*). The significance of this is that if the focal–film distance is doubled the mA-s output of the X-ray machine has to be quadrupled to compensate for this. Therefore low output X-ray units can only be used at comparatively short focal–film distances (usually not more than 75 cm). The practical application of this law in selecting exposure factors will be considered further in Chapter 7.

The effect of positioning

The positioning for specific examinations will be dealt with in Part 2, but the theory of the *geometry of image formation* must be mentioned here because factors such as *magnification* and *distortion* do materially affect the detail and definition of the image.

The X-ray beam like visible light, obeys the laws of central projection. The rays diverge from their source in straight lines and any interposed object will cause an enlarged 'shadow'. The simplest example is the light from a candle shining on to a white wall. If a hand is interposed a shadow will appear on the wall. When the hand is close to the wall, its shadow will be approximately the same size as the hand with crisp outlines, but as the hand is moved backwards towards the candle, the shadow will become increasingly magnified and diffuse until the image becomes unrecognizable. From this follows one of the basic rules of radiographic positioning—*place the part to be radiographed as near to the film as possible*. The magnification and loss of detail which occur when this is not possible is exemplified when attempting to radiograph the lateral lumbar spine of the adult horse or bovine.

In this examination it is not possible to place the vertebrae close to the film because of the interposed soft tissues. To demonstrate the effect of magnification on detail, a radiograph of a dried vertebra is reproduced in Fig. 3.4. In the live animal complications such as variable tissue thickness and the build-up of secondary scatter also degrade the image. The dried bone was radiographed (*a*) laid on the cassette, and (*b*) 30 cm above the cassette—the approximate object–film distance in life (Fig. 3.3).

Fig. 3.3   Magnification due to object–film distance.

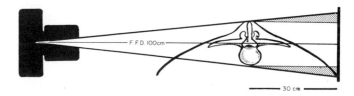

F.F.D. 100cm

30 cm

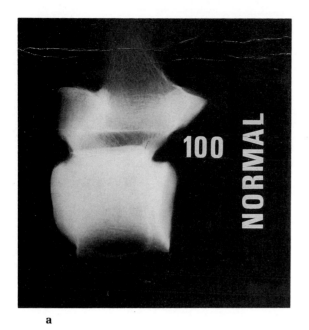

a

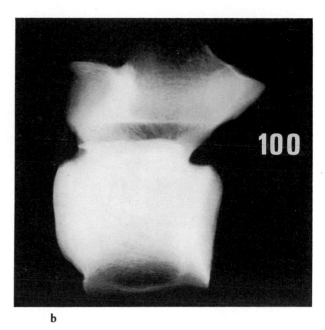

b

Focal–film distance and magnification

A focal–film distance of 100 cm was chosen for the radiography of the equine lumbar spine above for two reasons:

1 The average focussed stationary grid operates at this distance.
2 A greater distance would require an increased exposure which would be excessive, even for a high-power unit.

In order to reduce the magnification it is theoretically desirable to increase the focal–film distance to 180 cm because at this distance the rays reaching the film are virtually parallel. Conversely, a reduction of the focal–film distance to 75 cm increases the magnification and loss of detail when the part under examination is 30 cm from the film (Figs 3.5 and 3.6).

The effect of focal spot size

If the origin of the X-ray beam—the tube focus—were a true point source, simple magnification due to object–film distance would

Fig. 3.4 Note the magnification and loss of detail in (b) compared with (a).

Fig. 3.5 Variations in magnification due to changing the focal–film distance.

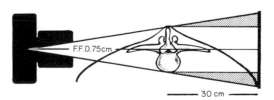

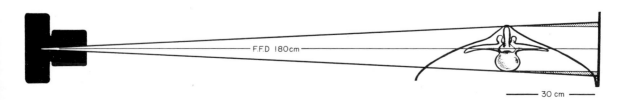

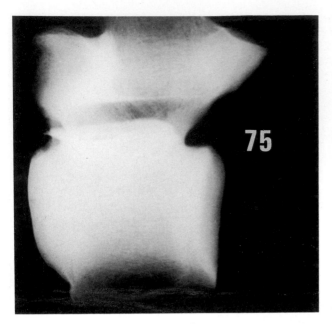
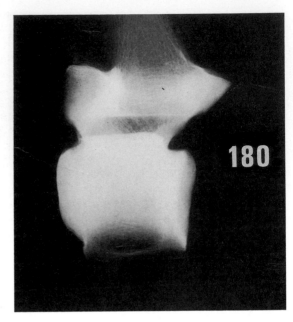

Fig. 3.6   X-rays—75 cm F.F.D. and
180 cm F.F.D.

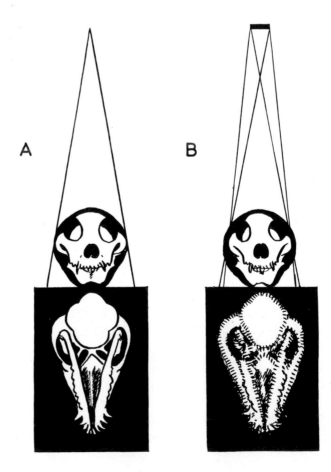

Fig. 3.7   Diagram to show the effect of
focal-spot size. In A the spot is a pin-point
and the projected image is sharp. In B the
rays from a focal-spot of large dimensions
cause a penumbral effect which blurs the
projected image.

not cause any loss of sharpness of the image. Unsharpness (or loss of detail) is caused because every focal spot has definite dimensions, usually covering an area of between 1 and 2 mm^2, and X-ray photons arise from all over this area. As explained in Chapter 1 all focal spots represent a compromise between the ideal pinpoint size required to produce maximum definition in a radiograph and the larger area necessary to withstand the heat generated when the anode is bombarded with electrons in order to produce X-rays. As the object–film distance is increased, the effect of focal spot size on the image becomes apparent. A penumbra or halo is formed which blurs the outlines of the densities and thus reduces both detail and contrast (Fig. 3.7).

The degree of unsharpness depends upon the same factors that govern magnification. As the size of the focal spot is a constant in most small units, any enlargement of a structure due to magnification will be accompanied by loss of sharpness.

Distortion

The concept of the central ray is an important one in radiographic positioning; it represents the centre of the area of radiation and the *point of minimum distortion.* A simple fact, which should never be forgotten is that the X-ray beam diverges. If the beam is not correctly centred, the ray traversing the region under examination will be at an angle and the resulting image will be distorted.

Accurate centring is most important when radiographing joint spaces; the canine stifle is a good example (Fig. 3.8). (For full details see p. 169). The hind limb is first correctly aligned on the cassette. The central ray is directed through the joint space at right angles to the film. An error in centring of as little as 1 cm

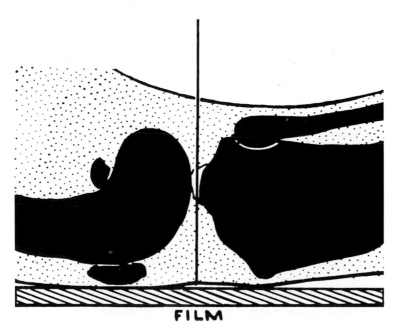

FILM   Fig. 3.8

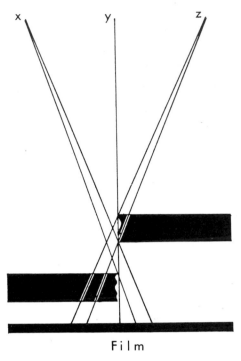

Fig. 3.9

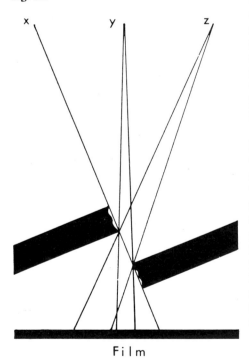

Fig. 3.10

can result in a distorted image—the femoral condyles will be superimposed on to the head of the tibia and it will not be possible to make an accurate radiological assessment of the joint.

Off-centring can also complicate the assessment of fractures, especially where there is separation of the fragments.

When the fragments of a bone lie parallel with the film (Fig. 3.9) but with vertical separation, the correct centring point y will show the fracture but not the displacement. If the tube is off-centred to z the peripheral rays will cause the image to show overlapping of the fragments. At x, the fragments will appear to show separation. When the fragments lie obliquely to the plane of the film (Fig. 3.10), the correct centring point y will distort the separation and so allowance must be made for this if a fractured bone appears foreshortened.

The distortions which can occur emphasize the desirability of always taking two views.

SCATTERED RADIATION

Up to this point it has been assumed that when a photon of radiation enters tissue or other structures, it either penetrates right through or is completely absorbed in the process. This is only partly true. While these are the two principal effects of the complex interaction of the X-ray photon with the atomic structure of the material penetrated, there is a third effect which can be of considerable importance. This effect is the production of *scattered radiation*. The generation of scattered radiation, as discussed in Chapter 1 (p. 17), essentially comprises the production, within the tissue irradiated, of new X-ray photons which are of longer wavelength than those of the primary beam and which emerge from the area penetrated in all directions (i.e. they no longer follow the path of the primary beam) (Fig. 3.11).

The scattered radiation produced by exposures made at the lower kilovoltages is of little significance because it is of long wavelength, has little penetrating power, and is very largely absorbed by adjacent tissues. At higher kilovoltages, particularly when radiographing very thick and dense areas of tissue, the secondary radiation produced is of shorter wavelength and is scattered from the tissues irradiated. This emerging radiation presents a safety hazard to persons restraining an animal for radiography (see Chapter 6) and, because it has not travelled in a straight line, results in blurring of the image produced in the film. Unless steps are taken to reduce the effects of scattered radiation, radiographs of the spine and abdomen of the larger dog and of most areas of the horse can be so spoilt as to be useless for diagnostic purposes.

The limitation of scattered radiation

The largest amount of scattered radiation is produced, and poses the greatest problems, when kilovoltage factors in the higher

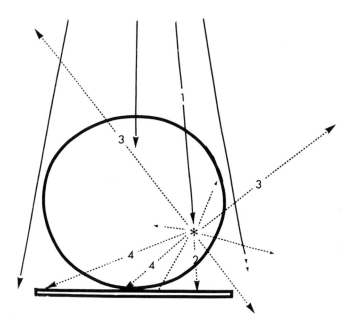

Fig. 3.11 Scattered radiation. 1: A primary ray which is scattered in all directions. 2: Some scattered rays aid in image formation because they travel in the same direction as the original primary ray. 3: Many scattered rays have sufficient power to pass outside the body and constitute a radiation hazard. 4: Rays which travel obliquely to the primary beam will degrade and fog the film. (Some scattering is, however, absorbed within the body.)

ranges are employed in order to permit penetration of the thicker and denser areas of tissue. In these circumstances the production of scattered radiation cannot be completely avoided but its effects can be minimized by reducing the amount of tissue penetrated, by preventing back scatter, and by using a grid.

Reduction of the amount of tissue penetrated by the primary beam

As described on p. 37 the X-ray beam should always be collimated in order to restrict the area of the patient which is actually traversed to the minimum necessary for the investigation.

When radiographing the abdomen the thickness of the part can also be reduced by using a compression (or Bucky) band (Fig. 3.12). This is a simple and effective way of reducing the depth of abdominal tissue of fat animals and it also helps to check the effect of respiratory movement and to restrain the patient. All X-ray manufacturers market this device, and although it is designed for standard X-ray tables, it can easily be modified to fit a veterinary examination table.

It consists of a band of cloth, 20–30 cm wide, which is placed across the patient and hooked into place on one side of the table. The other end of the band fits into a roller on the opposite side of the table. The band is tightened across the animal by turning the roller; tension being maintained by a pawl. Experience has shown that in most instances even the conscious dog will tolerate the use of this device.

The major disadvantage of compression is that it distorts the natural relationship of the organs within the abdomen and may

Fig. 3.12   Compression band.

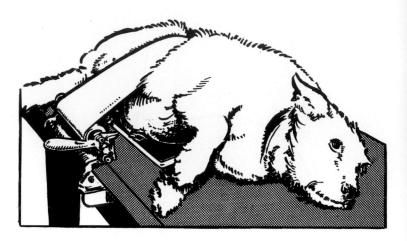

make diagnosis difficult. Obviously it should not be employed if there is any risk to abdominal organs (e.g. uterus or urinary bladder).

When a compression band is not available, several wide bandages can be passed over the animal and around the table to compress the abdomen, but this is a cumbersome expedient.

Prevention of back scatter

Scattered radiation is produced, not only when the primary beam passes through the patient, but also if the same beam having traversed the film, reaches the underlying table. Such scattered radiation, arising immediately adjacent to the film, could be a significant cause of blurring of the film. For this reason film cassettes normally contain a thin backing of lead, but when using high kilovoltages this should be reinforced by placing a sheet of lead or lead-rubber beneath the cassette and if film is used without a cassette (e.g. envelope wrapped non-screen film) similar precautions should be taken.

The use of a grid

A grid is a flat plate, about 2 to 4 mm in thickness, made in the various film sizes. It is constructed of fine strips of lead which alternate with strips of radiotranslucent material, either plastic or aluminium. In use the grid is placed immediately on top of the film cassette, but it is better to incorporate it into a special holder to protect it from damage. The grid acts as a filter and only allows radiation travelling in the line of the primary beam to pass through to the film below. Secondary radiation hitting the grid from other directions will be absorbed by the lead slats.

There are several forms of the *stationary grid* which is the type of grid usually employed for veterinary purposes (Fig. 3.13).

Parallel grid

In the parallel or linear grid the slats are parallel to each other and at right angles to the surface of the grid. They are not of such

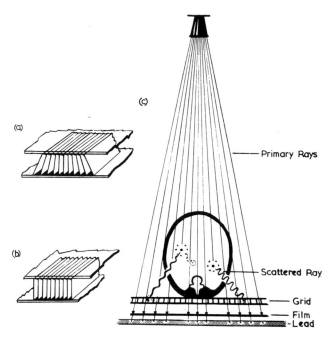

(c)

(a)

(b)

Primary Rays

Scattered Ray

Grid

Film

Lead

Fig. 3.13 (a) Section of focussed grid; (b) section of parallel grid; (c) the filtration effect of the stationary grid.

intricate construction as the other types of grid and are, therefore, slightly cheaper. They have the disadvantage however, that when used at short focal–film distances, the outer diverging portions of the primary beam tend to hit the lead slats and and are absorbed rather than passing between them. This is likely to result in significant under-exposure of the edge of a radiograph (grid cut-off) unless a focal–film distance of approximately 150 cm can be employed (this will not be possible with low power apparatus).

Focussed grids

Here the slats radiate. In other words, beginning from the centre long-axis, the slats on either side are progressively inclined at a greater angle to allow for the divergence of the peripheral rays of the beam. Such grids are manufactured to be used at particular focal–film distances (e.g. 75 cm, 100 cm or 180 cm) but they do allow some latitude and slight variation from the focal–film distance recommended for a particular grid will not significantly impair the standard of the radiograph. Precise positioning of these grids is, however, important. Obviously they must not be placed upside down and the central ray of the primary beam must always be aligned to the long axis of the grid. If the grid is displaced to one side the radiating slats will impede the primary beam and the resultant radiograph will be underexposed.

A grid is needed most when attempting to penetrate thick areas of tissue in large animals. Unfortunately in these circumstances the grid is often obscured by the bulk of the animal and it can be extremely difficult to align it precisely with the primary beam unless some additional device is available to assist with accurate centring.

Pseudo-focussed grids

This is a compromise between the two types already described. Since the construction of a precisely focussed grid is an extremely difficult process, some manufacturers prefer to concentrate on producing a perfectly uniform parallel grid and to overcome the absorption of primary radiation at the edge of the beam by a progressive reduction in the height of the lead strips (Fig. 3.14).

Fig. 3.14   Section of pseudo-focussed grid.

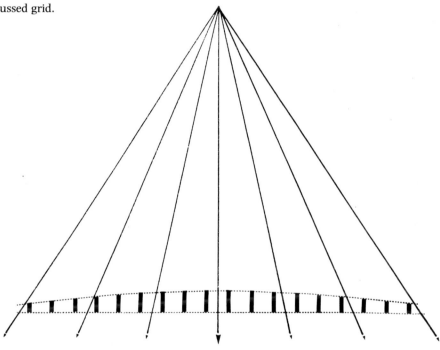

Crossed grids

Two parallel or focussed grids are set precisely at right-angles to each other and to the primary beam in order to achieve maximum filtering of scattered radiation in both directions. Centring must be very accurate or significant grid cut-off will occur. This type of grid is only necessary when the kilovoltage exceeds 100 (e.g. when radiographing the equine lumbar spine) and a large amount of scattered radiation is produced. The use of crossed grids is not practicable unless a means of aligning the primary beam very accurately with the grids and cassette is also available.

The Potter–Bucky diaphragm or moving grid

This device (Fig. 3.15) is used extensively in human work and in most large veterinary institutions in conjunction with large apparatus. Its value lies in filtering scattered radiation while eliminating the grid lines from the film.

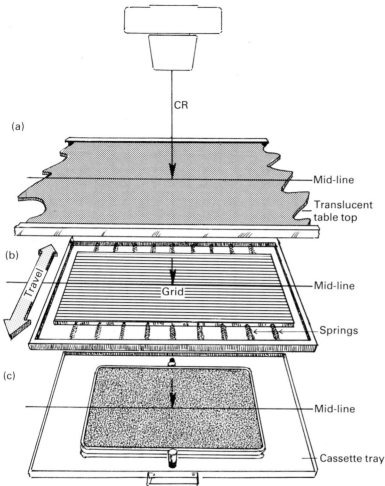

Fig. 3.15 The essential components of a Potter–Bucky diaphragm.

The diaphragm consists of a focussed grid which is moved mechanically across the beam of X-rays at a uniform speed—the rate of travel being adjusted to the exposure time. Advanced designs use reciprocating or catapult mechanisms to allow very short exposure times to be used.

The 'Bucky' is usually fitted underneath the X-ray table or in a vertical wall mounting. It cannot be used easily with small portable units, although many mobile machines do have suitable connections.

The grid factor is in the order of 4.

Grid efficiency

The efficiency of a grid in reducing scatter depends upon its construction. The number of lead slats to the centimetre, the width of the slats in relation to the width of the radiotranslucent material, and the thickness of the grid, all affect its performance.

Grid factor

Inevitably the lead slats will absorb some of the photons of the primary beam and the exposure must be increased to compensate for this. The amount the mA-s must be multiplied to allow for absorption (usually 2.5 to 3) is termed the *grid factor*.

Lines to the centimetre

It is important that the lead slats, or lines, should be barely detectable on the radiograph. Coarse slats would obviously break up the radiographic image. The number of lines to the centimetre, found in different grids, varies. The average number for medium kV work is 24. Very fine grids are made with 40 lines to the centimetre; they are almost invisible on the radiograph but unfortunately they are expensive and are designed mainly for high kV work, (i.e. 80 to 150 kV) and require very precise positioning (24 and 40 lines to the centimetre = 60 and 100 lines to the inch).

Grid ratio

The height of the lead strips in relation to the spacing between them is given as a ratio, such as 8 : 1, 10 : 1, 16 : 1. The greater the grid ratio, the more selective it is in allowing radiation to pass. This will significantly raise the grid factor.

Care of the grid

Grids are delicate and expensive items. If they are dropped on to their edges, they may be irretrievably damaged. Deep cassettes can be purchased to special order which have a recess in the front to house a grid and are called *grid cassettes*.

Cassette tunnel

A grid can also be mounted in the roof of a cassette tunnel which will allow a number of cassettes to be exposed without changing the film each time in the dark room (Fig. 3.16). In constructing such a tunnel care must be taken to see that the grid is closely applied to the cassette.

Purchasing a grid

A veterinary surgeon intending to purchase a stationary grid may be offered a wide range from which to choose. He should bear the following factors in mind:

1   *Expense.* These are expensive pieces of equipment. They are, however, essential if one is to obtain good quality films of the spine, pelvis or abdomen of the larger dog, and of the thicker regions of the horse.

2   *Size.* It is a false economy to purchase a small grid and then to find it necessary to subsequently purchase a larger one. For

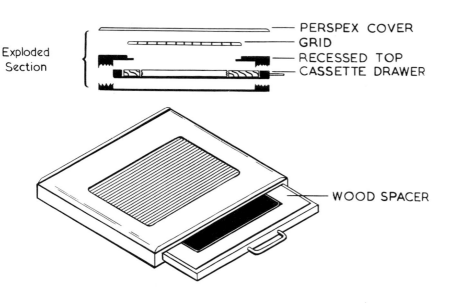

Exploded Section

— PERSPEX COVER
— GRID
— RECESSED TOP
— CASSETTE DRAWER

— WOOD SPACER

Fig. 3.16 Cassette tunnel.

small animal use the grid should not be less than 24 × 30 cm, but for equine navicular work 18 × 24 cm would be suitable.

3 *Type.* A focussed grid is most suitable for use at the short focal–film distances which have to be employed with lower output X-ray apparatus. It does, however, have to be more accurately positioned than a parallel grid.

The cheapest grids which incorporate wide lead slats and a low grid ratio are of very limited usefulness, while those with a particularly high grid ratio will have a high grid factor, require particularly precise positioning, and are extremely expensive. A grid intermediate between these extremes is suitable for most veterinary purposes.

4 *Grid Factor.* The use of a grid will always involve increasing the exposure factors. For veterinary purposes this factor should not be higher than 2.5 or 3 and even this may necessitate anaesthetization of the patient to prevent movement during the longer exposure times which are required.

5 *Grid Ratio.* A grid ratio of from 5 to 8 is suitable for most purposes.

SUMMARY OF SCATTER LIMITATION DEVICES

Scatter cannot be completely eliminated. In cats and small dogs, its effects are negligible, providing:

1 The beam is collimated to the precise area under investigation (e.g. if a survey film has revealed evidence of a lesion in the urinary bladder, this will be demonstrated more clearly by coning down to that organ, rather than by taking further radiographs of the whole abdomen).

2 After taking all other exposure considerations into account, the kilovoltage is kept as low as possible.

With larger dogs:

1   A collimation device, preferably a light beam diaphragm, is essential.

2   Compression may be applied to the abdomen, unless contra-indicated by the patient's condition.

3   Use rare-earth intensifying screens which are less responsive to low-energy scattered radiation than the older type of screen.

4   The use of a grid is usually recommended for tissues which are more than 10 cm in depth but remember that, unless the grid is correctly positioned, it may hinder, rather than assist, the production of a good radiograph.

5   Lead-rubber should be placed under non-screen film envelopes to absorb back scatter.

Wilhelm Roentgen produced the first medical radiograph shortly after his discovery of X-rays in 1895. A hand, which is generally believed to be his wife's, was placed on a glass photographic plate contained in a light-tight envelope and exposed to the new rays. This produced a full-sized image of the internal structure of the hand and this technique is still preferred for diagnosis, even though other, more economical, methods based on recording from an image on a fluoroscopic screen by cine, miniature film or videotape, have been developed.

It soon became apparent that the photographic emulsions available at the time were not ideal for capturing the X-ray radiant image, their sensitivity being mainly for visible light at the blue end of the spectrum. This necessitated the early X-ray exposures being unacceptably long, especially for veterinary applications. In 1852 Stokes had demonstrated that a number of substances possessed the property of absorbing electromagnetic radiation of a certain wavelength and instantly re-emitting it at a longer wavelength (i.e. as visible light). It was this fluorescent property of barium platinocyanide which had led to the subsequent discovery of X-rays. In 1896 Thomas Edison and others demonstrated that it was possible to reduce the exposure time for radiographs to more reasonable levels by converting the few photons of high energy in the X-ray beam into many photons of low energy—but longer wavelength (blue light)—by passing the beam through a layer of crystals of calcium tungstate. When this theory was transformed into commercial reality, two *intensifying screens* were used to sandwich a special double-coated X-ray film. Each screen consisted of a layer of carefully graded crystals of calcium tungstate mounted on a cardboard base and closely pressed against the photographic emulsion coatings in a light-tight container termed a *cassette*. The use of this combination reduced exposure time dramatically and greatly extended the scope of radiographic investigations. These essential accessories (intensifying screens and cassettes) will therefore be described before discussing X-ray film in greater detail.

INTENSIFYING SCREENS

An intensifying screen consists of a number of layers on a plastic base. Immediately above the plastic material there is a white reflecting surface, then a uniform coating of the phosphor and finally the whole is covered with a thin waterproof protective layer (the supercoat). Two screens are used inside a film cassette to sandwich the X-ray film, which is coated with emulsion on both sides, in close and uniform contact.

The range of screen phosphors

Materials selected for use in intensifying screens should possess three main properties:

1 They should have a high absorption coefficient and be able to absorb X-rays to a considerable degree. For this reason most substances selected have a fairly high atomic number.

Chapter 4

Recording the X-ray Image

2   They should emit a large amount of light of a suitable energy and colour.

3   There should be no significant *afterglow* (continued emission of light after irradiation of the material has stopped).

Accordingly, zinc cadmium sulphide, which fluoresces strongly with a yellow-green light, has been used for fluoroscopic screens since this is the part of the spectrum to which the human eye is most sensitive. Similarly calcium tungstate and, to a less extent, zinc sulphide, have been employed in the manufacture of intensifying screens because they emit light in the ultraviolet-blue end of the spectrum, to which photographic film is most susceptible.

Calcium tungstate has been the phosphor of choice for many years because of its even response over a wide range of kilovoltages. In the early days natural crystals were used which were large, uneven in size and suffered from afterglow. Now carefully graded artificial crystals are used and their speed has been enhanced by the incorporation of sensitizers.

It has been known for many years however that the rare-earth group of compounds could theoretically provide an even more efficient utilization of the X-ray beam but there were considerable difficulties connected with their purification for use. These problems have been resolved as a by-product of space research and now they are widely marketed and have become the standard screen phosphor for medical radiography.

Rare-earth phosphors have two main advantages over conventional calcium tungstate. Firstly, they absorb a greater proportion of X-ray photons and secondly they are more efficient at converting them into light. Thus, rare-earth screens make better use of the available X-ray photons and produce more light without any reduction in image quality. The reduction in the amount of radiation required to produce radiographs comparable with those using calcium tungstate allows the use of shorter exposure times (thus decreasing movement blur) and can extend the capabilities of low-powered apparatus. Image quality is improved despite the increased speed of these phosphors and their use reduces both personnel and patient dosage.

The rare-earth phosphors currently in use include:

1   *Lanthanum Oxybromide.*   This is a blue light emitting compound which can be used with those X-ray films that are normally employed with calcium tungstate screens. Examples of manufacturers who market such screens are Agfa-Gevaert with their 'S.E.System' and Dupont with the 'Quanta' range.

2   *Gadolinium and Lanthanum Oxysulphide.*   These phosphors are predominantly green light emitters and so require special (orthochromatic) film to be used and this in turn entails the use of dark-red safe lights. Manufacturers include 3 M with their 'Trimax' system and Kodak with the 'Lanex' series.

Screen material

In the production of intensifying screens the manufacturers attempt to combine two essential properties—*speed* (the smallest possible exposure) and optimum *definition* of the radiographic image. Unfortunately those factors which contribute to either one of these attributes tend to have a deleterious effect on the other and so a compromise has to be reached, depending on the purpose for which the screen is intended.

Speed is increased by making the phosphor layer thicker and by incorporating sensitizers in it. However the light produced tends to diffuse through the greater thickness and causes loss of definition or *screen unsharpness*.

Definition is facilitated by thin layers of crystals and by the inclusion of certain impurities which check the diffusion of light through the phosphor layer (but also prevent as much light reaching and affecting the X-ray film).

In most circumstances the advantages of reducing the amount and time of exposure are more important than obtaining perfect definition and, unless the fastest screens are combined with the fastest films, the slight loss of detail is not of great significance. In veterinary radiography speed of exposure may in fact contribute to better definition by eliminating the effects of uncontrollable movement of the patient.

Screen speed

There are a large number of intensifying screens marketed and their comparative value in intensifying the diagnostic X-ray beam is usually indicated by the use of one, or both, of the following terms.

Intensification factor. This is calculated by dividing the amount of exposure required when screens are not used by that necessary when screens are used. The figure may vary with the value of the kilovoltage and other factors, but it is likely to range from approximately 35 for the slowest (high definition) screens to 200 for the fastest rare-earth screens.

Speed. Most manufacturers produce a range of three screens and, instead of comparing them with exposures without screens, they quantify them in relation to the rest of the range. The most frequently used 'standard' screen is considered to have a speed of one. The speed of faster screens (which need less exposure) is rated as a fraction of this (usually 0.5) and that of slower screens as a multiple of 1 (usually 1.5 to 2). However one manufacturer's range of screens will seldom be exactly like another—nor will one generation of screens be comparable with another. For example, a standard rare-earth screen may be twice the speed of a standard calcium tungstate screen and still give the same image quality.

Note that these two scales for assessing intensification are *inversely* related to each other (i.e. the higher intensification factors correspond with the lower speed measurements).

Range of screens

As already mentioned the basic range of screens made with a specific phosphor will usually consist of three types:

1 *Standard.* Also referred to as 'normal', 'regular' or 'par-speed'.

These will consist of a carefully balanced blend of crystal size (5µm), dyes, sensitizers and coating thickness to give good resolution (e.g. of the canine abdomen) at an acceptably low exposure level.

2   *High definition (fine grain).* These are ideal for examinations which require optimum detail and where exposure time is of less importance—particularly for bone work when voluntary and involuntary movement can be controlled. Exposure usually has to be increased by a factor of 1.5 to 2. Rare-earth high definition screens are roughly equivalent in speed to standard tungstate screens but have a far higher resolution.

Some manufacturers aid resolution further by incorporating a dye in order to reduce the lateral diffusion of light which is a major cause of blurring, and this tints the phosphor surface.

3   *Fast or High Speed.* When the overriding concern is to reduce exposure time or patient dosage, or to penetrate a very thick area of tissue, fast screens can be used, but at the cost of increased grain in the image. This graininess is due mainly to light diffusion through the thicker layer of crystals, rather than the inclusion of larger crystals.

The increased speed of rare-earth screens has also led to an effect appearing termed *quantum mottle* or *radiographic noise.* This is a spotty or mottled appearance which is not due to grain size, but is due to the fact that the screens are so sensitive that only a few photons are necessary to produce an X-ray image of the correct density. These few photons however do not pattern the area in an even manner and have been likened to the first spatterings of large raindrops upon a pavement. When greater exposures are needed this effect is evened out and is no longer perceptible. Quantum mottle is a major disadvantage of the use of rare-earth screens for very brief exposures, but its effects can be mitigated by the right combination of films and screens.

The care of intensifying screens

Screens are expensive and easily damaged. An unnoticed splash of developer, or a knock which causes an abrasion of the surface, will permanently damage the screen, and an artefact will be present on all films taken in conjunction with that screen. It is not unknown for a wrong diagnosis to be made from a radiograph bearing an unsuspected artefact.

Dust and animal hair are also constant nuisances which should be regularly removed with a soft brush, as they will cause extraneous shadows on a radiograph by blocking the transmission of light to the film.

The supercoating can be cleaned by careful swabbing of the surface with dampened balls of cotton wool and good quality soap. Rinse off the soap using very little water, before standing upright to dry in dust-free room. If a proprietary screen cleaner in an aerosol can is used, spray on to cotton wool or tissue, rather than on to the screens. Proprietary cleaners have the advantage of possessing antistatic properties. At all other times the cassettes should be kept closed to prevent accidental damage. Never touch the screens with the fingers and never write on a film still in the cassette.

FILM CASSETTES

A cassette (see Fig. 4.1) is a light-tight container which is designed to hold the X-ray film and intensifying screens in close contact. Special cassettes will also hold a stationary grid as well.

The smooth face is termed the front and is made of material which is opaque to light but is radiolucent to X-rays—aluminium, plastic or, more recently, carbon fibre. The front is usually marked out into quadrants to allow more than one exposure to be made on the same film by masking off with lead rubber strips. An area about 7 × 3 cm may also be marked off in one corner to warn of the presence of a lead blocker inserted to prevent irradiation of the part of the film used for patient identification. Such details will be recorded by means of a light marker (see p. 90) but care must be taken to see that vital areas of the patient are not placed over this part.

The hinged back of the cassette is of heavier material and bears the catches which keep the cassette tightly shut. They should be examined in the light to see how they operate because some of them are difficult to open in the dark.

When the cassette is opened it will be seen that the inside is lined by the two phosphor-bearing surfaces of the intensifying screens. The front screen is mounted directly on the inside of the front panel and the rear screen on a pressure pad that ensures that film and screens are in close contact. The back plate of the cassette is also normally lined by a thin sheet of tin-lead foil to prevent back scatter from fogging the film. When using penetrating exposures for heavy animals this shielding should be augmented by placing the cassette on a piece of lead-rubber.

Cassettes, screens and films are made in various standard sizes to correspond with each other. In Britain and Europe these dimensions are now metric.

The veterinary radiographer should always look for cassettes of sturdy construction with good catches (e.g. ones which close effectively but are easy to manipulate in the dark) as they have to endure heavy usage.

Mounting intensifying screens in the cassette

Intensifying screens should never be loose, but must be properly mounted into the cassette. Because certain adhesives interact with the screens it is advisable to use only the double-sided tape provided by the manufacturers.

Some screens are marked FRONT and BACK and should be placed appropriately. In such instances the front screen will have been made slightly thinner so that it does not absorb an excessive amount of the X-ray beam and render the back screen less effective. In practice this precaution does not appear to be very important and many screens are of equal thickness and are interchangeable.

To mount a pair of new screens, first remove the protective layers from the tape mounted on the back of the screen and drop it carefully into the front well of the cassette with the fluorescent surface uppermost. Then place the second screen over it, but

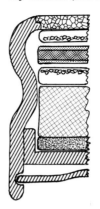

Fig. 4.1 Exploded section through an X-ray cassette (not to scale).

Radiolucent front
Front screen
X-ray film
Back screen

Pressure pad

Lead backing
Hinged backplate
Clip

upside down, so that the two fluorescent surfaces are in contact. Strip off the protective layers of the tape and close the cassette. The normal pressure will cause the screens to stick firmly, but leave for 24 hours to make sure.

The care of cassettes

1   Do not drop them on a hard floor. If this results in any loss of the close contact between film and screens, areas of unsharpness will be produced on the films and their diagnostic value may be impaired.
2   Do not trap the edges of the screens when the cassette is closed.
3   Cassettes should be kept clean, and there is always the danger of blood or urine leaking to the inside of the cassette. When a cassette must be placed in a dirty situation, put it in a plastic bag.
4   If more than one type of screen is used, mark the outside of the cassette to indicate the type of screen within.

Check for screen contact

Cassettes, particularly those which have been roughly handled, should be checked regularly by examining the films produced in them for any evidence of poor screen contact or of light leakage. The latter will be recognized as areas of blackening around the

Fig. 4.2a   Good screen contact.

Fig. 4.2b   Poor screen contact.

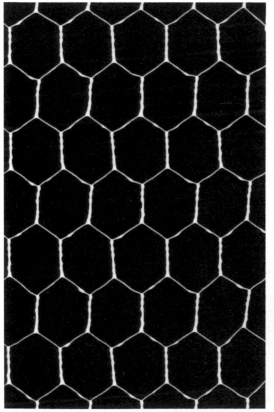

Fig. 4.2a

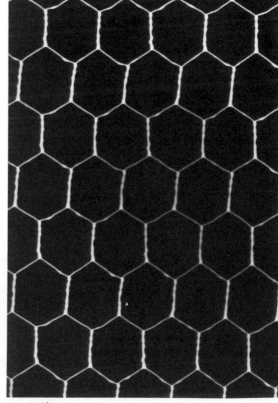

Fig. 4.2b

edge of the film, but a slight loss of contact, producing a reduction of definition, can be difficult to evaluate and can be best demonstrated by carrying out the following test:

1   Place a sheet of perforated zinc or flat wire mesh in close contact with the front of the loaded cassette.
2   Make a relatively light X-ray exposure (e.g. 45–50 kV and 3 mA-s at 90–100 cm FFD).
3   Develop the film as usual.
4   Examine the dry film for evidence of loss of screen contact which will be shown by areas of fuzziness of the pattern of the metal grid and increased density (blackening) of the small circles representing the holes in the grid.

X-RAY FILM

If an undeveloped X-ray film is examined in daylight (see Fig. 4.3) it will be found to consist of a support base of polyester plastic coated on both sides with thin layers of apple-green or fawn photographic emulsion.

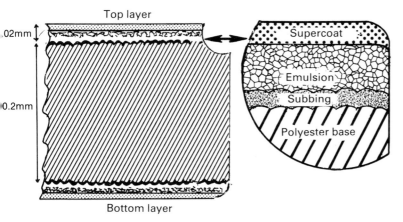

Fig. 4.3   Section of X-ray film, showing emulsion coats bound to the base by subbing layers and protected by supercoats.

Emulsion

Note that the base is coated *on both sides* by emulsion. X-rays pass through the film with minimum absorption and both layers are exposed simultaneously. This gives greater sensitivity to the film, doubling speed, density and contrast. Theoretically this effect would be the same if the emulsion were in one thick layer, but intensifying screens could not be used so effectively and the processing chemicals would take longer to penetrate the emulsion.

The emulsion of an X-ray film consists of a special gelatine containing finely dispersed minute grains of silver halide (usually silver bromide). The formulation of the emulsion is simple in principle but technically most complex. Silver nitrate in solution is added to a solution of potassium bromide and iodide in warm gelatine. In the interaction a precipitate of insoluble silver halides is held dispersed in the gelatine and the unwanted potassium nitrate and iodide are removed by washing.

The precipitate in the jelly subsequently undergoes a number of processes which determine the character of the emulsion e.g.

grain size, speed and spectral sensitivity, before it is coated on to the base.

The characteristic curve

The characteristics of an emulsion are usually expressed as a graph termed a 'characteristic curve' and are based on sensitometric data, the quantitative measurement of photographic density produced by a known exposure, for a specified time.

For X-ray films the emulsion is exposed to a beam of radiation which has been passed through a stepwedge. Each step is individually calibrated so that the exact amount of radiation passing through it and affecting the film can be calculated and thus provide a series of exposures. For convenience, the exposure values are then converted into logarithms and plotted against the baseline of a graph (the log-exposure axis).

The exposure value results in a degree of blackening of the test film—called *opacity* and caused by the conversion of the silver halide into metallic silver. Density is the common logarithm of opacity and is quantified by measuring the light falling onto a film (incident light—*I*) and the light passing through it (transmitted light—*E*). Density is then expressed as a logarithm of the ratio between the two

$$\text{Density} = \log_{10}\frac{I}{E}$$

The densities obtained from the series of exposures are plotted against the vertical axis of the graph, and the resulting line obtained from the data is an S-shaped curve (Fig. 4.4).

The points of interest are:

a The line always begins above zero, even without exposure. No processed film is completely transparent and this opacity is termed *basic fog*. It should be as low as possible and usually lies in the region of 0.1–0.3.

b The *toe* of the curve is where the exposure begins to have a visible effect on the film, and is just measurably greater than the fog level. The range of densities represent the 'bright' regions of a radiograph as might be seen in an area of dense bone.

c The *straight line portion* of the graph. A large portion of the characteristic curve is a straight line and is where the density of the photographic image is in direct proportion to the differences in brightness of the object. This part of the curve is also referred to as the region of *correct exposure*. The gradient of the straight line portion is termed the *gamma* and gives a measure of the speed and latitude of the film under test.

d The *shoulder* of the curve is where the effect of increased exposure has a decreasing effect upon film density. This corresponds with the very darkest parts of a radiograph, as may be seen outside a patient when the X-ray beam has not been sufficiently collimated.

The *gamma* is the tan of the angle (α) of the slope of the straight portion of the characteristic curve. It is a measure of the relation between density and the log exposure. When gamma is at unity

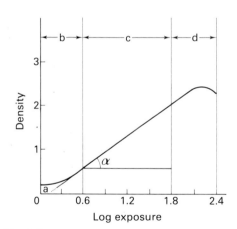

Fig. 4.4

(i.e. when the angle of the slope is at 45° to the log. exposure axis) then all the image densities will be directly proportional to the differences in log. exposure. At less than unity the image will appear flat and lack contrast. More than unity will give an image of greater contrast between tones but a shorter range of greys, so when the line is nearer vertical the image has great contrast and a 'soot and whitewash' appearance.

In photography, film speed is derived from the sensitometric data and various systems have been devised to use it for exposure calculation, e.g. H. & D., Scheiner, DIN etc. It is not practical to use such systems for X-ray work because in practice the curve changes at each different level of applied kilovoltage. Nevertheless, the characteristic curve does give the user much valuable information regarding *speed*, *latitude* and *contrast*. This is demonstrated in Fig. 4.5, showing the characteristic curves for two different films.

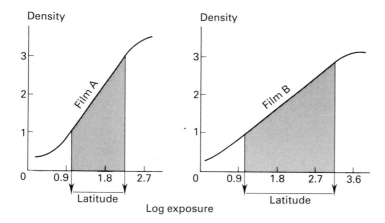

Fig. 4.5

Film A has greater speed than B (it requires less exposure to X-rays to produce the same degree of blackening of the film). It also demonstrates a steeper slope or higher gamma of the characteristic curve. This means that film A produces more contrast and less latitude than B and will therefore require more precise selection of exposure factors. Latitude is the range of exposures which will produce an acceptable density on the film.

Types of screen film

Films are manufactured to correspond with a certain range of intensifying screens and care must be taken to match them—especially the new range of rare-earth screens because of their specific range of light emission.

Films are also made in various speeds, in broad terms, slow, medium or fast, but these are often marketed euphemistically as 'high detail', 'par-speed' and 'ultra-speed' respectively.

Slow films (high detail)

This category is characterized by having a very fine-grained emulsion coated thinly and enabling fine detail to be demonstrated. In general they possess a wide latitude to exposure, long storage time and a resistance to basic fog. To aid high resolution some manufacturers add a coloured dye to the subbing layer (between the base and the emulsion) to reduce lateral disperal of light (e.g. 3M's 'Trimax XUD'). Such films are very suitable for extremity examinations and for the lung fields of cats and small dogs. Improved detail is however gained at the expense of speed and exposures will be 1.5–2 times those for standard films.

Medium speed films (standard or par-speed)

This is the category most widely used by veterinary surgeons and represents the compromise between fine-grain and speed. It is suitable for a wide range of examinations and so will often be the only type of film stocked in veterinary practice. The speed is rated as ONE and acts as the standard by which manufacturers rate the other films within their range.

Fast films (ultra-speed)

Although improvements in emulsion performance are being made all the time, it is still true that the fast emulsions have less exposure latitude, are more susceptible to background radiation and have a shorter shelf-life than the slower types. They also have a higher level of basic fog. They are of value when it is of paramount importance to use the shortest possible exposure—e.g. chest examinations in conjunction with low-powered X-ray units.

As already mentioned, the use of fast films *and* fast screens is not recommended because of the appearance of quantum mottle and grain.

Films for special purposes

Direct exposure or non-screen film

This special film, supplied in light tight envelopes, was used for many years to record the fine detail of the extremities and similar areas without the aid of intensifying screens. A thicker layer of emulsion was required as the effect of the X-ray beam was no longer 'intensified' but it overcame the slight loss of definition associated with the use of some of the coarser screens. Unfortunately the increased thickness of such film necessitated a longer processing time and it was not suitable for use in automatic processors. The manufacture and adoption of fine-grain films and screens has now led to the withdrawal of such films (e.g. Kodak 'Kodirex') which require manual processing. Some manufacturers do make a direct exposure film which can be processed manually or automatically and is useful for intra-oral studies where thick cassettes cannot be inserted. An example is 3M's Type S film. Exposures are very long, but the superior resolution allows much finer detail to be visualized in the image. However, it is useless for soft tissue work.

Kodak manufacture a direct exposure film designed for industrial purposes which is useful for morbid specimens only and which must be processed manually (Kodak 'Industrex CX').

Copy film

Occasionally it is desirable to make copy radiographs direct from the X-ray film. This is now very easily achieved using X-ray duplicating film, which has a special reversal emulsion. The original and copy film are placed together in a printing frame and exposed to white light in the same manner as making ordinary contact prints. The copy is then processed normally.

X-ray screen film with a blue dye image

'Medichrome' is an X-ray screen film marketed by Agfa-Gevaert in which, after processing in a special developer, a blue-coloured image is produced in a similar manner to colour transparency photographic film.

The main advantage claimed for this film is that the translucency of the image allows the contrast to be varied by viewing the radiograph through different yellow filters and that this allows the radiologist to concentrate on either bony or soft tissue detail in the same radiograph. In addition, the virtual lack of grain allows a fine rendering of detail and some radiologists find a blue image easier to view than a black one.

However, the film requires an increased exposure and very precise maintenance of developer temperature (a variation of 0.5°C or more results in a marked loss of film quality). At present the film is also more expensive than conventional films.

Single layer emulsion film

A medium to high contrast film with a single coating of high-definition emulsion, designed to be used with a fine rare-earth *single* intensifying screen for recording very fine detail.

The 'Polaroid' instant X-ray system

Polaroid-Land are well known for promoting instant dry photography, based on the *diffusion transfer reversal process*. They have now marketed a 'Polaroid' Instant Radiographic System which enables a radiograph to be produced, without a conventional dark-room, in the field within minutes of being taken.

The resultant image is a positive, blue-tinted transparency (unlike the usual radiograph which is a negative). For commercial reasons the only size available at present is 20.3×25.4 cm (8×10 in).

The equipment for the system comprises a special film cassette containing a single rare-earth screen, a very small portable film processor and loading tray and the film—Polaroid-Land Type TPX.

The film has two major components—a *light sensitive* negative film in a light-tight envelope and a transparent blue-tinted polyester imaging (or receiving sheet) which is *chemically sensitive*. The pods of processing chemicals are attached to the second sheet.

It is upon the imaging sheet that the X-ray image is viewed. The negative component is not readable or reusable and is scrapped after processing.

Details of the procedure involved when using this system to make a radiograph are explained and summarized in Fig. 4.6.

a   The X-ray latent image is recorded on to the negative component of the Polaroid-Land TXP film in the usual way but using a special cassette with a single rare-earth intensifying screen.

b   The imaging sheet (the second component of the film) with the attached developer pods is placed in the loading tray and the exposed film is placed over it. The tray is then inserted in the processor where the pods of chemicals are ruptured and the two components of the film are brought into close contact by the action of the rollers.

c   The developer not only converts the latent image on the negative to metallic silver but also acts on the unexposed silver halide to release free silver atoms. These diffuse to the imaging plate

Fig. 4.6

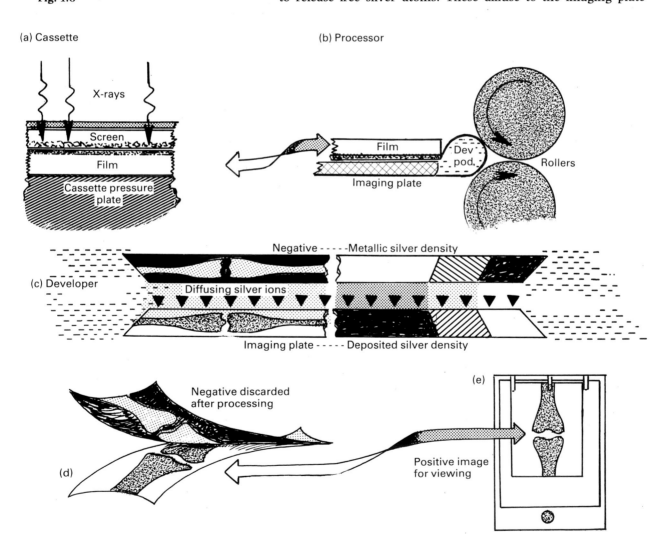

(a) Cassette

(b) Processor

(c) Developer

(d)

(e)

which is chemically receptive and form a black metallic deposit. The density of the deposit on the imaging sheet is in inverse relationship to the blackening on the negative, i.e. it is a positive image.

d After processing, the imaging sheet is peeled away from the negative which is discarded.

e The imaging sheet is a transparency and is viewed on a viewing box in the normal manner.

The processor can be operated manually or electrically. In the latter instance an audible signal is given on completion of the processing cycle.

For long term storage the positive film requires coating with a protective polymer which is supplied with each packet of film.

Although considerably more expensive than conventional film, the Polaroid system is of value—especially for equine domiciliary visits.

Film sizes

The dimensions of the different sizes of X-ray films vary from country to country. British manufacturers have changed from imperial to metric measurements, which involves cassettes, intensifying screens, hangers and radiographic equipment, as well as films. The sizes in general use are:

$$13 \times 18\,cm$$
$$15 \times 30\,cm$$
$$15 \times 40\,cm$$
$$18 \times 24\,cm$$
$$20 \times 40\,cm$$
$$24 \times 30\,cm$$
$$30 \times 40\,cm$$
$$35 \times 35\,cm$$
$$35 \times 43\,cm$$

Film packaging

X-ray film suitable for veterinary work is packaged in three main ways

Folder wrapped

In this type, each film in a box is covered in a folded sheet of yellow paper. The paper is not lightproof so the box must be opened only in a darkroom. The paper is also useful as a cheap filing folder for dry films.

Boxes usually contain 50 or 100 films.

Bulk-packaged film

This type of pack is intended for the larger volume user and films are not covered by yellow paper folders. Usually sold in 100 and 500 packs.

Envelope wrapped film

A convenient form of packing for direct-exposure films which can be used straight from the box. The film is wrapped in a paper folder enclosed in a stout, lightproof envelope with a cardboard stiffener.

Usually packed with 25 envelopes in a box.

Unexposed film storage

If films are kept for a long period in an unsuitable place, storage fog will develop. Sensitive materials should be stored in a cool, dry room away from strong chemical fumes. If they are kept in a room adjacent to the X-ray room, the wall or cupboard should be lined with lead of 1.5 mm thickness (or material of the lead equivalent) for voltages up to 100 kV.

In tropical or hot, humid climates, the films are best kept in cold storage until shortly before a box is required. After opening, a box of films should not be put back into cold storage.

Film emulsion is sensitive to pressure, so film boxes should be stacked on end in the store. Where there is a good delivery service, do not keep a large stock of films. Write the date of arrival on the boxes so that they are used in the correct order.

THE X-RAY IMAGE

The development of the latent image in an exposed X-ray film is considered in the next chapter. Nevertheless, it is appropriate in this chapter, to consider the qualities which should be present in the radiographic image when it is finally visualized by correct processing.

A radiograph should be inspected for technical quality after it has been developed and fixed. Technical quality is difficult to define because there are so many interrelated factors, but the main consideration must be whether or not the film is a *diagnostic* radiograph. Is the area under examination sufficiently visualized to solve the clinical problem for which it was taken?

A radiographer must know when a film is technically bad, and *why*, so that the fault can be corrected. Because many factors influence the formation of the image, a certain amount of practical experience is necessary, since the appearance of the X-ray image can be deceptive. For instance, an overpenetrated film of an extremity can show anomalous translucencies in the bones which can be mistaken for osteolysis, dried splashes of developer on an intensifying screen can cause an artefact on the film similar to a calculus, while superimposition of bone fragments has frequently masked a fracture.

Qualities of a diagnostic radiograph

The requirements of a good diagnostic radiograph are:

1   An accurate portrayal of the structures under examination, i.e. good *positioning* with the minimum of geometric distortion.

This has been considered in Chapter 3 and will be implicit in much of Part 2 of this book.

2 Easy perception of the relevant structures. The quality of both the *contrast* and the *detail* should be good.

3 There should not be any misleading *artefacts*.

Contrast

Contrast is defined as the numerical difference between two adjacent densities. In more practical terms, it is the degree of perceptible difference between two tones (Fig. 4.7). An image of a white bone against a solid black background with no intermediate grey tones

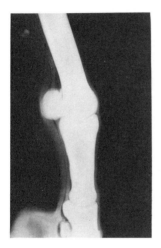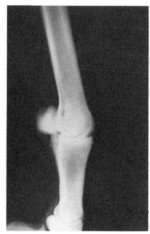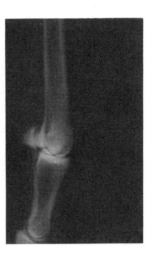

Fig. 4.7 Left to right: high, medium and low contrast.

is described as having *high* contrast. A *flat* film, on the other hand, containing no blacks or whites but only tones of grey has *low* contrast.

Neither of these extremes is desirable. A good radiograph should have a long range of well differentiated densities so that the eye can easily see the detail.

The common cause of poor contrast lies in the choice of exposure factors.

Exposure factors

Kilovoltage affects both contrast and density. If it is too *low* the resulting film will have a 'soot and whitewash' appearance, i.e. high contrast. When the kilovoltage is too *high*, contrast will be reduced because the shorter wavelength X-rays will more easily penetrate bone and other dense tissues and lower the contrast which should have been produced by the differential absorption of soft and dense structures. Some radiographic examinations, particularly those of the canine chest and of the equine pedal bone, rely on this property of high kilovoltage to overcome the excessive contrast which otherwise would be seen in radiographs of these areas.

The mA-s Factor (milliamperes × time) affects film density by governing the amount of X-ray photons which reach the film emulsion. This, however, only affects film contrast in a negative way, by reducing the contrast when the mA-s factor is incorrect. If the quantity of X-rays reaching the film is too low, the film will be pale. Close inspection will reveal that dense structures have been penetrated, but by insufficient photons to build up a satisfactory image. Overexposure will cause increased overall densities so that very little transmitted light from a viewing box will be allowed to get through.

Distance affects contrast only when it is altered without compensating the mA-s factor.

X-ray film contrast

Film manufacturers carefully prepare X-ray film emulsions to produce good contrast under optimum conditions and the veterinary user will find that all the reputable brands, irrespective of their speed, will give satisfactory results if used correctly.

Intensifying screens increase image contrast and screen-film emulsions are formulated with this in mind. Non-screen films have a higher contrast than screen films.

Processing

Apart from incorrect exposure, the most common cause of poor film contrast is bad processing. This can be due to development at too low a temperature or for too short a time, or to incorrect replenishment or exhaustion of the developer. Over-development can increase contrast slightly but is not recommended.

Fog

Veiling of the image by fog results in lower contrast because the 'highlights' are degraded. A certain amount of fog is inherent in all types of emulsion and is termed *basic fog*, but this should not exceed a density level of 0.2. The fog level can be raised by several factors:

1 Premature exposure to white light, bad safe-lighting or X-rays.
2 Secondary radiation.
3 Excessive development by time or temperature ('processing fog').
4 Overlong storage or storage in hot, humid conditions.

Detail and definition

The details of an X-ray image depend for their perceptibility upon their contrast with the background and upon their definition, or sharpness.

The concept of contrast and its effect upon detail has been dealt with in the preceding section, but two points should be mentioned. First, very small details need high contrast if they are to be easily seen. Secondly, when one density merges gradually into another (a contrast gradient) the eye will find it difficult to perceive the difference. If the two densities are separated by a firm line of demarcation, the difference can easily be seen. Definition is ruined if the film image is blurred.

A certain amount of blurring is intrinsic in any radiograph, due to such factors as the size of the focal spot, intensification screen grain size and the lines of the stationary grid. These can be minimized only by the careful choice of apparatus, but they do not affect the diagnostic image in veterinary radiography to any appreciable extent, in comparison with the effects of the extrinsic factors: movement and magnification.

Magnification and other geometric effects have already been discussed. The results can only be noted but rarely controlled with small apparatus. Movement is the most common cause of lack of definition, and it should be minimized.

Artefacts

The film image is often marred by artefacts caused by dust in the cassette, screen marks, faulty processing, etc. A list of the commoner causes is given at the end of this chapter. Apart from indicating an oversight in the radiographic routine, they lead to misdiagnosis. If a mark consistently appears on films, the cassette should be isolated and the screens examined and cleaned. If the fault is persistent but easily recognizable, the front of the cassette should be marked 'Faulty Screens', but if the damage could lead to misdiagnosis the screens should be replaced.

Areas of poor definition may be caused by poor screen contact. The fault may be corrected by judicious packing, but if it remains persistent the cassette should be scrapped.

Occasionally, a small fault in the film emulsion may cause uncertainty about whether it is an artefact or a lesion in the patient. This can often be determined by examination of the surface of the emulsion by reflected light.

Viewing the radiograph

Radiographs should be viewed on a good, evenly-lit viewing box, in a semi-darkened room. Because image contrast depends upon the intensity of the light transmitted through it, many viewing boxes are fitted with dimmer switches to enable the light to be varied. It may be noticed that a detail may often be more clearly seen when looking at the film from the side than from the front. This is because the transmitted light must pass through a slightly thicker section of the film and the light is slightly reduced in intensity, thereby enhancing the contrast of the detail.

Contrast can be improved by holding a dense, relatively over-exposed part of a film against a bright tungsten electric light bulb. Some viewing boxes incorporate a 'Photoflood' lamp for this purpose.

When a small film is mounted on a large viewing box, the bright light from around the edges will cause the pupils of the viewers' eyes to contract, making the retinas less sensitive to the subtle contrasts of the much dimmer light transmitted through the film. Masking the bright edges with black cardboard greatly improves detail perceptibility.

Although a provisional diagnosis must usually be made on a wet film, it is advisable to wait until the film is dry before finalizing a diagnosis which depends upon the elucidation of fine detail, because when the film is swollen with water, the transmitted light is refracted to a certain extent. The individual emulsion grains are also spread out when swollen. When dry they contract together and so increase definition.

Viewing a radiograph

Veterinary radiographers generally follow the medical convention of viewing radiographs of the dorsoventral chest or ventrodorsal abdomen or skull with the right side of the film facing the viewers' left side.

Radiological diagnosis

The assessment of radiographic quality must precede any attempt at diagnosis because confident interpretation is impossible from poor film.

Good radiological interpretation must not only be based on visual evidence but on the data from a comprehensive physical and clinical examination of the patient. The practitioner must have knowledge of the range of radiological animal anatomy; and here a 'library' of normal films taken in the standard positions for comparison is an asset. Interpretation begins with the examination of the outlines and density of the detail, but this is where the subject of radiography becomes radiology and is beyond the scope of this book.

Table 4.1   Film faults

Defect	Cause
Film too dark	(a) Over-exposure (reduce kV or mA-s). (b) Gross overdevelopment time. (c) Developer temperature too high. (d) Excessive fog (see below).
Film too pale	(a) Under-exposure (increase kV or mA-s). (b) Developer time too short. (c) Developer temperature too low. (d) Developer exhausted. (e) Developer too diluted.
Faulty contrast High ('soot and whitewash')	Insufficient penetration (kV) of the dense portions of the subject.
Low (flat film)	(a) High kilovoltage. (b) Underdevelopment. (c) Excessive fog (see below).

Defect	Cause
Poor detail (unsharpness)	(a) Object–film distance too long. (b) Uneven screen contact in cassette. (c) Movement of apparatus or patient during exposure. (d) Coarse stationary grid lines. (e) Lack of grid.
Fog	Fog is an additional density, unconnected with the primary image, which reduces contrast and detail.

Generalized fog	(a) Storage fog.
	(b) Chemical fog, caused by gross overdevelopment.
	(c) Radiation fog, due to:
	  (1) Pre-exposure to ionizing radiations.
	  (2) Excessive secondary radiation (use grid, smaller field and reduce kV).
	(d) Light fog, due to wrong filter in safe-light or prolonged inspection during development.

Localized fogging at edges	Light penetrating into cassette, film box or film hopper.
Stained films, yellow stain Colour (dichroic) fog	Insufficient rinsing or use of exhausted fixer.
Artefacts Streaking	(a) Lack of agitation. (b) Dirty processing hangers. Dried-in fixer residue will contaminate subsequent films. (c) Insufficient rinsing. (d) Drying marks.
Airbells (clear white spots surrounded by a ring)	Air bubbles on the surface of the film. (Avoid by occasional agitation of the film in the developer.)
Crimp marks (black or white crescentic shadows)	Caused by crinkling the film by handling with excessive pressure between the index finger and thumb. If the crease is done before exposure it may appear black or white; if before development, black.
Abrasion marks	Long, grey pressure lines caused by the film sliding across the floor when accidentally dropped.
Static marks (arborescent black streaks)	Exposure caused by the discharge of static electricity. Can be caused when pulling a film out of a box without a folder, in a dry atmosphere.
Developer splashes (dark black spots)	The splashes cause local prolonged development.

Defect	Cause
Fixer splashes (white spots)	Local reduction of the emulsion before development.
Screen marks	
(*a*) clear white specks	Dust between the screens.
(*b*) small areas of light density	Dried developer splash marks on the screens.
Fingerprints (dark or light)	Handling of the film with dirty, greasy or contaminated hands.
Grid faults	
Vignetting or grid cut-off (areas of peripheral under-exposure)	(*a*) Wrong focal-film distance which does not correspond with the grid radius.
	(*b*) Off-centring from midline.
	(*c*) Angling beam across the grid lines.
	(*d*) Reversing grid.
Quantum mottle	
Spotty or mottled appearance	The use of very low exposure values in association with sensitive rare-earth screens.

The other 14 chapters of this book are almost entirely concerned with the radiographic theory and practice necessary to record the internal structure and pathology of veterinary patients on X-ray film. This record cannot, however, be visualized and used as an aid to diagnosis until the film has been suitably processed in a dark room. The details of processing are described in this chapter but it must be emphasized that, unless dark room construction and technique are maintained at a high standard, processing can impair, or even ruin, the most carefully thought out radiographic examination, rather than bring it to its full fruition.

Although the broad photographic principles of processing a radiographic film remain the same, the technology of the process has changed and in the majority of human hospitals is now fully automated. While a small, but increasing, number of automatic processors are used for veterinary radiography, processing is still very largely done by hand, using either tanks or dishes to hold the chemical solutions. At the present time the majority of veterinary dark rooms depend on tanks for processing and this technique will be described in detail before considering the advantages and disadvantages of the alternative methods available to the veterinary radiographer (i.e. dish development and automatic processing). The occasionally used 'Polaroid' Instant X-ray System which enables a radiograph to be produced without using a dark room is described in Chapter 4 (p. 65).

Chapter 5

The Dark Room

The layout of the radiographic dark room

A room should be set aside as a permanent dark room, ideally with a floor area of not less than 2.6×2 m (8×6 ft). Although individual circumstances must dictate where a dark room is to be sited, the following points might be borne in mind:

1 The room must be capable of being made completely light-proof.
2 It should not be damp or subjected to extremes of temperature.
3 Water and electrical outlets should be provided.

Lightproofing is often more difficult to achieve than may at first be thought. Light-lock entrances are not usually practicable and doors must fit closely into their frames, against strips of felt or rubber where necessary. A bolt must always be fitted on the inside of the door to prevent it being opened at the wrong moment. Light entering under a door or through pin-hole defects in the blackout can cause appreciable fogging of films. This may not be appreciated by those whose eyes are not adapted to the dark and it is necessary to spend some 5 minutes in the dark room without any lighting, before checking for any such defects. Furthermore the amount of light leaking into a dark room may vary with the intensity of the light outside. Defects in the lightproofing may not be of significance if processing is undertaken in the evening and yet serious fogging of films can occur in the same dark room if it is used on a sunny day.

Windows can be completely sealed but it is desirable that they should be opened occasionally to let in air and sunshine. Lightproof roller-blinds running in 15 cm (6 in) channels are most satisfactory.

Adequate ventilation of the dark room is essential if the room is in continuous use. Ventilation holes should be properly baffled, and painted matt-black on the inside.

The walls should be painted white or cream using a good quality washable paint. The part of the wall around the developing chemicals should be further protected by ceramic tiles, Melamine plastics or (cheapest) an impervious paint which is chemical resistant, stain resistant and waterproof.

The ceiling should be painted white (avoid the use of water-bound paints as these may flake and fall on to the processing area) to act as a good reflecting surface for the safe-lighting.

The floor must be capable of being easily washed over and impervious to processing solutions. Suitable flooring materials are terrazzo, earthenware tiles in acid-proof cement, rubber, vinyl or composition tiles or heavy-duty linoleum. Concrete floors are attacked by photographic chemicals after a time.

Dark room equipment

There are two main work points which must be kept as far away from each other as possible. They are designated the 'wet bench' and the 'dry bench'.

Dry bench

The dry bench is where the cassettes are unloaded and recharged with fresh film. It must be impossible for splashes of developer to reach the dry bench surface. When the dry and wet benches must be accommodated side by side, as illustrated, a suitable partition must separate them.

The top of the dry bench must be large enough to accommodate the largest cassette in use when opened out. The top surface should be either of wood or linoleum. Plastic laminates are not recommended because they hold static charges of electricity which can cause marks on films. It is usual to store film boxes, especially those in current use, beneath the dry bench, either in a cupboard (protected if near an X-ray set) or in a film hopper. Compartments can be installed to take cassettes. A wastepaper bin is also an asset.

The processing frames should hang above the bench, each size on its appropriate bracket. There are two designs of processing frame—the channel type and the clip type. Each has its advantages and disadvantages. The channel frames (Fig. 5.2a) tend to retain fluids within the channels and, therefore, need careful cleaning to prevent chemical deposits from contaminating films, and the films must be taken out of them for drying. Clip hangers (Fig. 5.2b) overcome these faults, but are more fragile, the clips can scratch adjacent films during processing and they are liable to get into a tangle if they are carelessly stored. Clip hangers are most useful when a film drying cabinet is available, or for holding very large films, e.g. 43 cm × 35 cm, which are liable to fall out of the channel hangers.

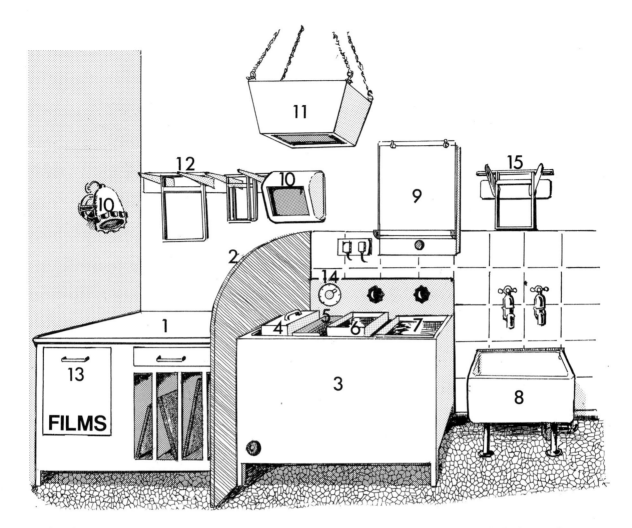

Fig. 5.1 A simple dark room layout.
1 Dry bench.
2 High partition between dry and wet benches.
3 Wet bench—manual processing unit.
4 Developer tank with lid.
5 Rinse water tank.
6 Fixer tank.
7 Wash tank.
8 Sink.
9 Viewing box.
10 Direct safe-light.
11 Indirect/direct ceiling safe-light.
12 Film hangers on wall rack.
13 Film hopper.
14 Thermostatic control and temperature gauge for processing unit water jacket.
15 Wall rack for wet hangers.

Wet bench

The wet bench is where the processing of the films is carried out. The usual method is to use a set of tanks holding developer, rinse water and fixer, and a larger tank for washing the films. The tanks can either be stood in a sink, when the developing solution will be warmed as required by means of an immersion heater, or they can all be placed in a thermostatically controlled water jacket. The latter is preferable and can either be purchased as a complete processing unit (several small reasonably priced units are available—Figs 5.3 and 5.4) or constructed by the handyman. For most purposes 9-litre (2-gallon, Imperial) tanks are suitable, but if they need to hold more than 3 films simultaneously, 22-litre (5-gallon) tanks will be necessary.

Tanks are manufactured in vulcanite, plastic and stainless steel. Vulcanite is the cheapest material, and tanks made from it give satisfactory service, although after long use they tend to bulge and increase their capacity and they can be fractured from rough usage. For this reason modern tanks are made from plastic or stainless steel. The washing tank should be at least four times

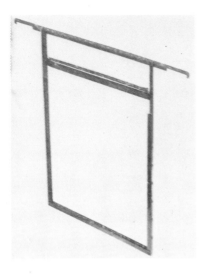

Fig. 5.2a   Ilford channel hanger.

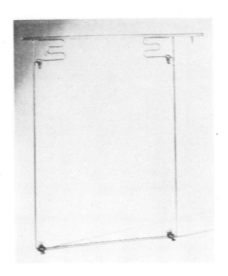

Fig. 5.2b   Ilford clip hanger.

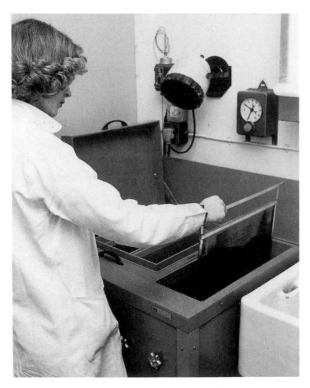

Fig. 5.3   A hand processing unit with 22 litre (5 Imperial gallon) capacity tanks: the PC Processing Unit. (By courtesy of GEC Medical Ltd.)

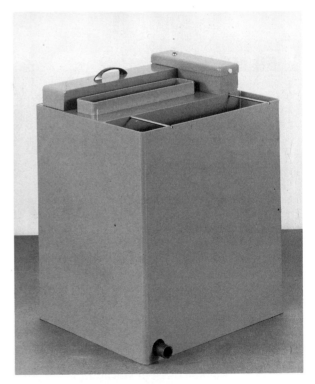

Fig. 5.4   A compact hand processing unit made of plastic. The developer and fixer tanks are of 13 litre (3 Imperial gallon) capacity. The Prefect Processing Unit. (By courtesy of PLF Medical Ltd.)

larger than the developer tank, with a supply of cold water circulating through it, via a rubber hose, when films are being washed.

Heaters and thermostats

Standardized processing requires that the developer is only used at the optimum temperature of 20°C (68°F) and this usually means that some heating of the solution before use will be necessary. It is possible to do this simply by having an immersion heater in the tank of developer and using it to raise the temperature to the required level. Unfortunately this method is time consuming in cold weather and, unless stirred carefully and checked, can still lead to development at too low or high a temperature.

The only satisfactory method for a busy practice is to use a method of heating which is thermostatically controlled and maintains the correct temperature so that the solution is ready for use at any time. This will involve either purchasing a processing unit or else constructing a suitable water jacket and fitting it with a thermostatic water heater. Heating of the tank containing the fixer solution is not essential, but if this can be contained in the same heated water bath it will prevent slowing of fixation in very cold weather.

In temperate countries the most important need is to have a means (as explained above) of raising the temperature of the developer to the correct level, but occasionally local climatic conditions lead to overheating and the reverse process is required. In very hot weather therefore it is advantageous to have a water jacket which is so fitted that fresh water from the mains may be circulated through it. Other emergency aids include the use of ice cubes in the water bath or electric fans in the dark room.

Ideally and for the best results, the developer solution should only be used at the correct temperature, but when this is impossible slight variations in the temperature can be compensated for by varying the time of development according to a chart provided by the manufacturers of the developer.

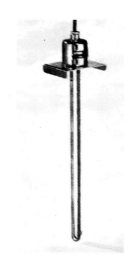

Fig. 5.5 Ilford X-ray tank immersion heater.

Tropical temperature control

It is very difficult to maintain the temperature of the processing solutions at the optimum of 20°C in those tropical countries in which the summer temperature is between 30°C and 40°C.

Where economic conditions permit, standards of film quality comparable to those achieved in temperate climates may be obtained by automatic processing in an air-conditioned environment or by the use of a refrigerated processing tank.

However in many tropical countries such facilities are not available and even water and electricity supplies may be restricted and erratic. The following points should be considered when attempting to ameliorate these extreme conditions:—

1 Only films made to the 'Rapid Process' (R.P.) specification should be purchased, as these are made to withstand high temperatures.

2   The X-ray developer formula should contain a hardener.
3   The developer temperature should be lowered by the liberal use of ice in the water jacket.
4   Processing times will be very short, but an attempt at proper 'time and temperature control' should be made by reference to the manufacturer's charts.
5   Fixing time should be increased to allow the hardener to function, as the emulsion will be very delicate and easily damaged.
6   Washing time can be shortened provided that a fresh supply is circulating. If water is restricted, a closed supply fed from a tank and circulated by a pump should be installed and fed through the wash tank. The use of a tank containing hypoeliminator to neutralize the fixer before washing will also aid in keeping down the level of water contamination, until such time as the supply of clean water can be renewed.

Drying

Films should always be removed from channel hangers before suspending them by a clip from a tensioned wire in an airy dust-free place (this may be outside the dark room). This process may take several hours, particularly in cold weather, and can be speeded up by using moderate heat (a hair dryer can be useful) or by purchasing a film drying cabinet.

Safe-lighting

X-ray film emulsion is very sensitive to white light before processing and can only be handled safely in a dark room illuminated by light of a specified colour and intensity. Essentially a safe-light is a box containing a low wattage bulb behind a suitable filter. There are two types which may be used in the radiographic dark room:

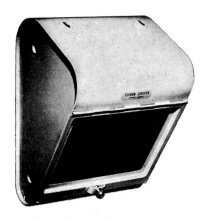

Fig. 5.6   Direct safe-light.

1   *Direct*—a diffused light shines directly over the workpoint, such as the dry and wet bench.
2   *Indirect*—the filtered light is directed up to the ceiling where it is reflected over the whole room. This is often combined with a direct safe-light.

Safe-light efficiency   Safe-lights should be placed so that the work of the dark room can be done without fumbling. Where the dry and wet benches are separate, a small direct wall light should be provided for each, and if the floor area exceeds 6 m² (60 ft²), a centrally placed indirect safe-light should also be provided.

The efficiency of the filtration may be tested by covering an unprocessed film with black paper or cardboard, placing it one metre from the safe-light and then uncovering portions of the film for periods of 0–10–20–30–60–120 seconds. No blackening of the film should be visible upon development. However no safe-lighting is completely safe if a film is placed too close to the light or for too long.

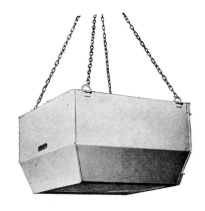

Fig. 5.7   Combined indirect (above) and direct (below) safe-light.

Safe-light filters   Blue sensitive (monochromatic) film which is used with calcium tungstate and some rare-earth screens needs a brown-coloured filter in direct safe-lights (e.g. Kodak Darkroom

Filter 'Wratten' Series 6B) and a light-brown filter for indirect safe-lights (e.g. Kodak Darkroom Filter 'Wratten' Series 6BR). Green sensitive (orthochromatic) film which is used with the other rare-earth screens requires a dark-red filter (e.g. Kodak Darkroom Filter Type GS-1).

PROCESSING THE X-RAY FILM

The routine of processing an X-ray film is a simple procedure which can be taught to any intelligent person in a short time. The exposed film is removed from the cassette in a safely lighted dark room and placed in a stainless steel processing frame. It is then immersed in a tank of developer which completes the reduction of the exposed grains of silver halide, and makes the image visible. After a specified time the film is taken out of the developer, rinsed in water and then immersed in the fixer bath. This solution removes the undeveloped halides. The image can now be inspected in white light. After 10 minutes in the fixer bath the film is washed in running water for half an hour, to remove the processing chemicals and then hung up to dry.

The most important point to be grasped is that the processing routine will be followed many hundreds of times, so continual care and cleanliness must always be observed to get optimum results. This is only possible if good dark room facilities are available. This does not necessarily mean costly apparatus but it does require the layout and fittings to be well thought out. Do not hesitate to write to the film manufacturers for advice. Do not economize and make do with a couple of dishes in an old washroom, except in an emergency. The resulting films will not be a credit to you.

The processing solutions

Consistent processing can be achieved only if standardized solutions are employed. X-ray developers and fixers should be purchased only from reputable manufacturers and used strictly according to their instructions.

The developer

An exposed film bears an invisible (latent) image of exposed silver ions. The developer solution converts these ions into minute grains of metallic silver.

$$Ag^+ \rightarrow Ag.$$

Development is most accurately described as a 'rate-selection process'. The developing agents first attack and reduce the exposed grains of silver halide, but after that they will begin reduction of the unexposed emulsion—causing development fog. There is, therefore, an optimum development time, which will vary from 3 to 5 minutes with different types of developer. When a new developer is being compounded, efforts are made to make the differentiation between the rate at which exposed and unexposed silver halide is reduced as wide as possible.

For many years the most efficient X-ray developer has been the metol-hydroquinone formula.

Metol (p-methylaminophenol) is a developing agent with a high reduction potential. It starts development rapidly and the whole image appears at the same time. Although detail is well rendered, the contrast of the image is low.

Hydroquinone has a low reduction potential and is very sensitive to temperature. It commences development slowly on the most heavily exposed portions of the image and produces high contrast.

When these agents are used together, they display the phenomenon of 'superadditivity', or a far better performance than the theoretical adding together of the results of separate development.

Phenidone (l-phenyl-3-pyrazolidone) is a new agent which is replacing metol as the partner of hydroquinone. It displays to an even greater extent the phenomenon of superadditivity, can be made up in greater concentrations and has a number of other advantages such as being able to work in the presence of bromine ions released from the film emulsion, which gives it a longer working life than metol.

Other ingredients in a developer solution include the alkali, the buffers to preserve pH, restrainers to maintain the developer's rate-selection capability, sequestering agents and hardeners.

The Alkali. Developers cannot function properly in an acidic or neutral environment. The greater the degree of alkalinity, the greater the activity of the developer. As an active developer is needed for X-ray work this is regulated at a pH of 10 or 11. The alkaline ingredient is termed the *accelerator* and for X-ray developers is usually a carbonate or hydroxide of sodium or potassium.

The Buffer. The pH of a developing solution is constantly being eroded during its working life by oxidation and other contamination. To preserve the correct degree of alkalinity, a chemical known as a buffer is added. This is an alkaline salt of a weak acid.

The Restrainer. Active developers not only attack and convert the exposed grains of silver halide emulsion to metallic silver but they also have a tendency to affect the unexposed grains, so producing a chemical fog which degrades the lighter portions of the image. The presence of bromine ions in the solution helps preserve the rate-selectivity and these are normally provided by the exchange between the developer and the film emulsion. A freshly prepared developer would lack these ions and so a restrainer (such as potassium bromide) is added initially, to act as a starter. Too many bromine ions would, however, inhibit the activity of the solution and so potassium bromide is omitted from the formula of replenishment developers.

Sequestering Agents. Hard water, if added to a concentrated alkaline developer solution, may result in a precipitate of calcium or magnesium salts occuring, and result in sludge and scale. Sequestering agents are included to prevent this as they have the ability to render sodium and magnesium salts soluble.

Hardeners. When films are processed at higher temperatures than the optimum of 20°C the gelatine of the film emulsion becomes swollen and soft and must be protected. Organic agents of the dialdehyde type are used for their hardening effect on the emulsion, but require careful control, or the action of the developer on the emulsion will suffer.

Types of X-ray developer

X-ray developers are marketed in powder and liquid forms. The latter is the simplest to use as it only requires dilution with the recommended amount of water before use.

The powder form is the cheaper and is only available for manual processing in dish or tank. It should not be prepared in the dark room as the inevitable chemical dust can cause contamination of unprotected films. It is better to make it up in a bucket outside the room before putting the mixture in the tank and diluting to the final working volume. For dish use the solution should be stored in dark bottles.

The optimum temperature of a working solution of developer is 20°C (68°F). Recommended development times vary with different formulations but are usually between 3 and 5 minutes.

Replenishment

Replenishment of the developer serves the double purpose of replacing lost volume and maintaining as far as possible an even activity.

A large film will absorb about 60 ml of solution, most of which will be carried over into the rinse water, no matter how long the film has been drained first. This lost volume obviously cannot be replaced by topping up with water. Chemical changes also occur in the developer after a number of films have been processed. These must be regulated because standardized processing cannot be maintained if the developer changes its characteristics during its working life.

Developer replenisher is a specially balanced solution made for adding to the developer to keep up the volume and maintain consistent characteristics. It is usually purchased in equal volume with the developer and then made up, by dilution, and stored in dark, stoppered bottles until required. The usual practice is to replenish to a volume equal to that of the original developer—for example, a 9-litre (2-gallon) tank of developer will absorb 9 litres (2 gallons) of replenisher. The solutions are then thrown away and new developer and replenisher made up.

Made-up solutions should never be kept for more than 3 months as they will oxidize and be unfit for use. The oxidation rate is delayed if a floating lid is used as well as a tank lid, or if the developer is kept in dark stoppered bottles.

In the authors' experience the commonest processing fault is the use of cold or exhausted developer, which leads to 'under-development' with consequent lack of contrast and definition. This is a serious fault and is likely to make it impossible for the radiologist to appreciate fine detail in the final radiograph.

The fixer

The fixing bath contains a solvent of silver halide, either sodium or ammonium thiosulphate. When a film is put in the fixer, the unexposed halide is dissolved, leaving the metallic silver image, which can then be viewed in white light.

The secondary function of the X-ray fixer bath is to harden the gelatin by means of a tanning agent to render it less susceptible to scratches. It also contains an acid buffer to neutralize any developer which may be carried over.

The clearing time (the time taken for the unexposed halides to be dissolved) depends on a number of factors:

1   *Emulsion thickness.* A screen type film will fix in a shorter time than a non-screen film.
2   *Temperature.* A warm solution fixes faster than a cold one. However, above 21°C (70°F) staining can occur and the hardening properties of the fixer are quickly lost.
3   *Exhaustion.* A load of dissolved silver halides in the fixer will retard fixation and hardening. The exhaustion rate is greater than that of an equivalent amount of developer. This is especially true of powder fixers. A fixer is exhausted when the initial clearing time is doubled.
4   *Agitation.* This can reduce fixation time by half as it removes the saturated fixer from around the film and brings in fresh fixer to attack the remaining silver halide.
5   *Concentration.* There is an optimum concentration for each type of fixer solution (usually 40 per cent) which clears a film more readily than a higher or lower concentration.

The composition of the fixer

Fixing Agent. Sodium thiosulphate is used chiefly in those fixers which are marketed in powder form, while ammonium thiosulphate is employed for the concentrated liquid fixers. The latter salt has the advantage of a longer lasting and more rapid action, but if a film is left in the solution for an excessively long time, it can begin to reduce the developed image. It can also cause troublesome stains if splashed on to clothing.

Acid. A weak acid (glacial acetic acid or sodium or potassium metabisulphite) is included in order to neutralize any alkaline developer which remains in the emulsion despite rinsing. It rapidly stops any further development and prevents developer oxidation products from staining the film.

Preservative. The thiosulphate fixing agents have a tendency to decompose in an acid medium and a preservative is included to control this. Sodium sulphite and sodium or potassium metabisulphite are all used for this purpose with the two latter substances fulfilling a dual role as acidifiers and preservatives.

Hardener. The hardening of the film emulsion, which has become softened and swollen in the alkaline developer, is most effectively undertaken in the fixer bath because of its acid environment. Chrome and potassium alum are used in the powder fixers for this purpose but, like some of the other constituents, do not have a very long working life. Aluminium chloride and sulphate are hardening agents which are more soluble and can therefore be used in greater concentration and so act more quickly and last for a longer period. They are found chiefly in the liquid fixers and, because of their speed of action and suitability for higher temperatures, are also included in the fixers used for automatic processing.

Buffer. The fixing bath receives relatively large volumes of alkaline developer and loss of acidity could lead to inefficient hardening and the formation of dichroic fog. Usually sodium acetate with acetic acid is used as a buffer to maintain the pH at the optimum level.

Types of X-ray fixer

X-ray fixer can be made up from packed powder chemicals or from a liquid concentrate. Some makes of liquid fixer bottle the hardener separately and this is added after the main solution is diluted. Special formulations are made for automatic processors.

Liquid fixer is more expensive than powder but it is far more efficient. However, when the solution has been in use for some time, if any is splashed on to clothing, a persistent brown stain will appear after the garment is laundered. The stains are caused by silver in the fixer solution and can be removed from the garment by applying a household silver solvent to the spots, followed by a rinse in cold water before relaundering. Keep the solvent away from stainless steel fittings.

Powder fixers do not stain clothing, but their life is shorter and the film clearing time is longer. Because of the contaminating nature of fixer dust, mix powder fixers with water outside the dark room.

Washing

Water performs a valuable photographic function, namely the removal of residual developer and fixer salts from the film which otherwise would attack the image and turn it yellow and faded in a few years.

Ideally the whole film hanger should be immersed in the wash tank, and the water introduced via a rubber hose to a blind-ended, perforated tube which lies diagonally across the bottom of the tank (Fig. 5.8). A good circulation of water is essential. Washing usually takes at least 15 minutes at normal temperatures [13°C (55°F) to 25°C (77°F)], timed from the introduction of the last film into the tank, but this time should be doubled if the film is to be kept for a long period.

In areas where the water is very hard, a scum can settle on films which leads to drying marks. Where this occurs, the films should be immersed in a wetting agent (e.g. Kodak 'Photo-flo' or Ilford wetting agent) before hanging up to dry.

Fig. 5.8   Cut-away diagram to show how a perforated pipe on the bottom of the wash tank, connected to a tap by rubber tubing, supplies an even flow of water over the surface of the film. The outlet is situated near the top.

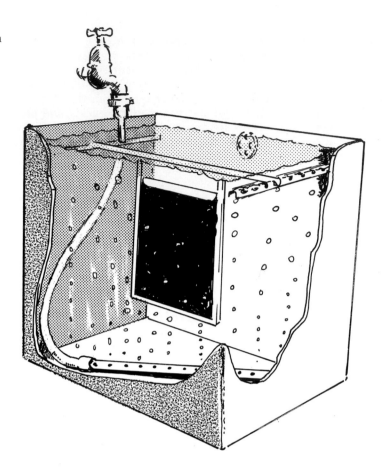

Processing of non-screen film

Because the emulsion of non-screen film is thicker, it takes longer for the processing solutions to permeate the film and reach the silver halides. The development time for these films should normally be increased by 1 minute and it will be found that clearing takes several minutes longer than with screen film.

Dish development

One of the main disadvantages of tank development is that, once made up and exposed to heat and air, the developer solution will deteriorate, even if it is only used very occasionally. The effect of this is likely to be appreciated after 2–3 months as a loss of radiographic quality and the only answer is complete replacement of the chemicals. This is rather wasteful, unless a sufficient number of films have been processed to justify the expense. Where only a small number of radiographs are processed annually, it is more satisfactory if small quantities of the processing solutions are made up as required, used in dishes and then discarded, rather than depending on stale solutions of unknown efficiency which have been kept in tanks for some time.

A much simpler dark room will suffice for dish development. The essential requirements are—complete blackout, a safe-light, a means of heating the developer, 3 large photographic dishes and a table to place the dishes on.

The solutions must first be made up to the correct working strength from either concentrated liquid or powder chemicals and the developer warmed to the correct temperature 20°C (68°F). The heated solution can cool rapidly in cold weather and it is helpful to place the dish on an electrically heated warming pad (marketed for horticultural and photographic purposes). Films of the sizes most commonly used can be processed in 30 cm × 25 cm dishes with about 1000 ml of each solution. Three suitably sized dishes are laid out on a table to contain the developer, rinse water and fixer.

The film is removed from the cassette and a small clip affixed to one corner. It is slid into the developer and the dish is gently tilted to keep the solution moving over the emulsion surface. Turn the film over frequently to prevent uneven development. When development is complete, rinse in water for a few seconds and then place in the fixer dish. Allow the fixer to clear the film evenly before inspecting it in white light. Finally wash the film thoroughly in running water.

Repeat the procedure for subsequent films, but do not process two films simultaneously. Discard the solutions after a few hours as the developer quickly oxidizes in open dishes and cannot be reused.

Because of the frequent use of freshly made up processing chemicals, development in dishes can produce better quality radiographs than by using tanks, but it is relatively more time consuming.

Automatic processing

Automatic processing of films has obvious advantages over the two methods just described. It saves time in the dark room, standardizes the processing procedure to a high degree and produces a dry radiograph ready for examination within a very short time (90 seconds with some machines). The cost of the necessary apparatus unfortunately precludes its routine use in veterinary practice, but the saving in labour hours and the convenience and consistent good quality of the radiographs could justify its installation in busy practices and clinics with a high radiographic throughput (small table-top machines can be purchased for around £2500–3500).

A dark room is still required to load and unload the film cassettes but the wet bench is replaced by the processor. An efficient dark room extractor fan must be fitted near the machine (Fig. 5.9a), because of the heat and fumes it produces when working. This problem is less acute when the major part of the processor protrudes through the dark room wall (Fig. 5.9b), but an extractor fan is still advisable.

Automatic machines follow roughly the same routine as manual processing, except that they operate at a higher temperature in order to speed development and the rinse between developer and fixer tanks is eliminated (the carryover chemicals are removed

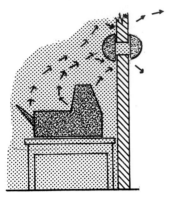

Fig. 5.9a

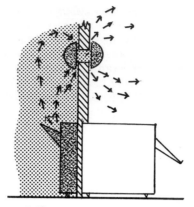

Fig. 5.9b

by compression as the films pass through squeegee rollers) (Fig. 5.10). In use, an exposed film is fed into the tray of the machine and is then transported through the chemical trays (or baths) and dryer by a roller assembly actuated by a worm drive. The solutions are kept in peak condition because fresh chemicals are introduced by a pump at a predetermined rate depending on film throughput. The temperature is also constantly monitored and controlled within fine limits.

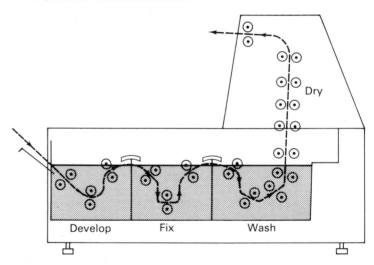

Fig. 5.10   The essential features of an automatic processor.

When operating a considerable amount of fluid will pass through the machine. Wash water is drawn from the domestic supply, which should be capable of delivering about 6 litres per minute, and in some models must be at a certain temperature (achieved by using a thermostatically controlled demand valve linked to the hot and cold supply). The unit must also be connected to an adequate drainage outlet for disposal of water and waste chemicals and, where the number of films processed justifies this, it can be linked to a silver recovery unit.

Operating routine

The manufacturers will supply detailed instructions for the care and operation of each machine, but this will usually involve:

1   Switching on the machine first thing each morning, as a variable (10–20 minutes) warm-up period is necessary before it can be left on stand-by and ready for immediate use for the rest of the day.

2   At the end of the warm-up period it is helpful to pass an old used film through the machine. This will confirm that it is functioning normally and will remove any chemical scum which may have accumulated on the rollers overnight.

3   When the day's work is finished, the machine should be switched off and those working parts of the processor which are exposed to the atmosphere and accessible should be wiped with a damp cloth to prevent a build up of chemical deposits. Do not use abrasive or chemical cleaners.

4   Once a week it is necessary to remove the rollers from the machine and to wash them in clean water. The levels of the processing chemicals should also be checked and topped-up if necessary.

5   Regular servicing of the apparatus by a suitably trained engineer should also be arranged.

Processing chemicals

Automatic development solutions are formulated for specific types of processors since these may operate at different temperatures or require different times to complete the processing cycle. The developer solution acts both as developer and as replenisher and, for this reason, when first introduced into the machine it is necessary to add a starter solution which reduces the activity of the 'developer-replenisher' to that of a normal developer. The fixing solution is suitable both for use in the processing tank and for replenishment.

Radiographic quality

As already mentioned, one of the main advantages of automatic processing is the *consistent* production of good quality radiographs. However, because of the high temperature at which development is undertaken there is a slight loss of the contrast and 'sparkle' which can be obtained when development is undertaken under ideal manual conditions (absolute cleanliness and freshly made up solutions) at the correct lower temperature 20°C (68°F). This optimum standard is, however, very difficult to maintain when hand processing and is most likely to be achieved when dishes are employed and fresh solutions are made up each time they are used.

Breakdown

As with all mechanical devices, automatic processors can break down, particularly if they have not been well maintained, and this is likely to cause serious inconvenience in a busy practice. In the event of a breakdown, service engineers will come as quickly as practicable, but it may be worth having the necessary chemicals and containers in store so that emergency hand processing can be undertaken if required.

Silver recovery

A relatively large amount of silver is lost in the waste material from automatic processors and it is possible to fit units designed to recover this to the waste pipe. Unfortunately such recovery is unlikely to be economic unless the number of films processed annually runs well into four figures. Silver merchants are usually very ready to advise whether this is practicable, and they may also be interested in purchasing old radiographs (again, if in large quantities) for reclamation of the silver they contain.

IDENTIFICATION OF THE RADIOGRAPH

It is helpful, and in some circumstances essential (e.g. when taking radiographs for certification under the hip dysplasia scheme), to have certain information incorporated in the radiograph, so that it is available when the film is examined subsequently. This may include:

1   Some means of identifying the particular patient.
2   The date of radiography.
3   An 'L' or 'R' to identify a particular limb or side of the patient.
4   Some indication of the time which has elapsed since the administration of a contrast medium.

This information may be added to the radiograph during radiography, during processing, or subsequently when the film is dry. Obviously the earlier the details can be attached to the film the less the risk of mistakes occurring.

Identification during radiography

The simplest way of carrying this out is by placing lead letters or numbers on top of the film holder (preferably fixed in place with Sellotape or similar radio-translucent material) before making the radiographic exposure. Another way of doing this is by using a specially prepared tape with radio-opaque backing on which information can be inscribed by writing or typing, such as X-rite tape, and then attaching it to the film cassette.

'L', 'R' and similar markers should always be added at this stage. If this information is attached to the film later it is only too easy to make mistakes in identifying a particular side of the patient.

Identification during processing

Essential information can be pencilled on a corner of the film in the dark room immediately before processing. Such identification is not very obvious or lasting and for long term purposes should be more permanently inscribed on the dried film before filing.

A more efficient method of identifying films is to use a light operated marker to print information photographically on a film. This device is usually mounted on the dry bench and the desired particulars are printed by a separate operation directly on to the

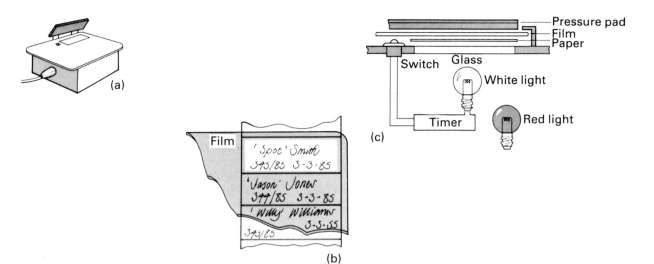

(a)

Film

'Spot' Smith
345/85 3·3·85

'Jason' Jones
344/85 3·3·85

'Willy' Williams
3·3·85
343/85

(b)

Pressure pad
Film
Paper

Switch Glass
White light
Timer Red light

(c)

film in a space which has been left unexposed by the incorporation in the cassette of a lead mask.

Identification of the dry film

Details can be entered directly on to the dry film either with a yellow 'Chinagraph' pencil, or, for a more permanent result, in white ink.

Any method of writing on the film is not a suitable method for marking films for the purpose of the hip dysplasia scheme or on any other occasion when 'legal' identification of a radiograph might be necessary. Printing the information on the film by either photographic or radiographic means is essential.

CARE AND STORAGE OF THE DRY RADIOGRAPH

The following notes on the care and storage of dry films may be useful:

1 Make sure the films are dry.
2 The practice of keeping films in their original paper protective folders from the film box is cheap, but less acceptable when many films are to be stored. It is more convenient to keep them in film storage envelopes.
3 Film envelopes can be filed either in a cabinet or on open shelves. It will be found that it is much easier to file films if all the envelopes are the same size.
4 Films of outstanding interest can be further protected by sealing them in polythene covers from which they need not be removed when handling and viewing.

DARK ROOM ROUTINE

Good dark room routine depends upon processing films under the standard conditions advised by the film manufacturers to produce the best results from their products.

Fig. 5.11 A light-operated film marker. (a) The unit can be free-standing or flush-fitted into the dark room dry bench. (b) A slip of paper bearing the patient's details, either typed or written in black ink, is placed over the glass panel and the film placed over it. The pressure pad is brought down to ensure good contact. This action also actuates an exposure of white light of predetermined duration. (c) A cross-section of the components of the marker.

Cleanliness

Walls, floors, benches, utensils and film hangers should be kept clean. Separate stirring rods should be kept for developer and fixer. The hands of the dark room worker should be rinsed and dried after touching the solutions.

Development time and temperature

It has already been mentioned that the optimum development time is 3 to 5 minutes and the temperature of the developer should be 20°C (68°F). Brief inspection of the developing film is permissible after 2 minutes if there is doubt about the correct exposure, especially when very small animals are being investigated. Underdevelopment will produce a reasonable film but not one of optimum quality, and should only be practised when overexposure is unavoidable. Overdevelopment can seldom improve an underexposed film. An extra minute may help, but it is also likely to increase the fog level. Modern developers are designed to produce optimum densities in a certain time and the best results can only be obtained by adopting a strict policy of time and temperature and, when necessary, correcting the exposure factors.

Frequent examination of the film during development may cause the formation of streaks or stains on the film surface. Close inspection near to the safe-light can also raise the fog level.

The X-ray film processing sequence

Preliminary

Check that the developer is at the correct level and temperature and has been stirred. Select the correct film hanger. Switch on safe-lights. Switch off white light.

Dry bench

Open the backplate of the cassette and gently shake the top well so the film can be grasped at its edge by the finger and thumb (Fig. 5.12). Use the light marker if available.

Loading the hanger

If a channel type hanger is used, hold it in the left hand and slide the film into the channels and close the top hinge (Fig. 5.13).

A tension clip hanger is loaded by inserting the film first into the bottom clips, then turning the hanger the right way up, insert the film into the upper spring clips (Fig. 5.14).

Identification

If it has not already been identified by photographic or radiographic means, the relevant information should be written in pencil on the top righthand corner of the film.

Close the cassette.

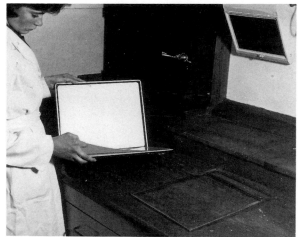

Fig. 5.12

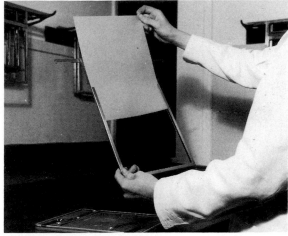

Fig. 5.13

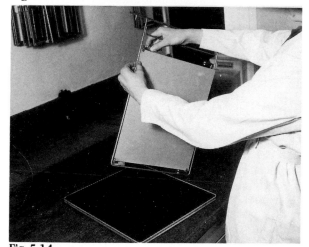

Fig. 5.14

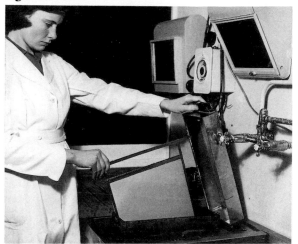

Fig. 5.15

Wet bench

Place the film in the developer (Fig. 5.15) and agitate two or three times to remove any air bubbles on the film surface. Place the lid on the developer tank. Set the interval timer. The film should be agitated further during development to remove the bromides released from the surface of the film during the chemical inter-action. In heavily exposed areas these released bromides can sink down preventing development of the parts of the film directly below and causing low density streaking.

If the hands are wet, rinse and dry thoroughly.

Reloading the cassette

Open the lid of the X-ray film box and extract a film in its folder by its edge. Film emulsion is sensitive to pressure, so do not fold or buckle film by careless handling.

Open the cassette.

Pull back the top leaf of the protective folder, twist the wrist and drop the film into the well of the cassette (Fig. 5.16). Withdraw

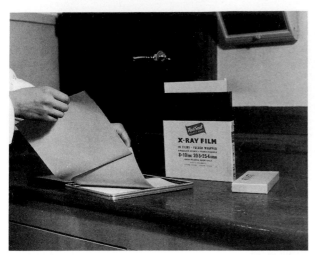

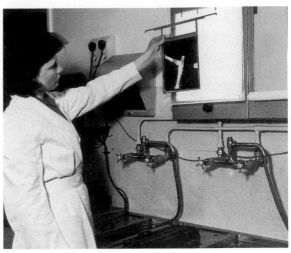

Fig. 5.16

Fig. 5.17

the folder. Run a finger around the edge of the well to make sure that the film is not protruding over the edge.

Close the cassette and replace the top on the film box.

At the end of the developing period, lift out the film and allow the solution to drain back into the developer tank for a few seconds.

Rinse in water for about 10 seconds.

Place film in the fixer.

Wait for 30 seconds.

The white light can now be switched on.

When the milky appearance caused by the dissolving silver halides has disappeared, the film can be viewed for technical quality and provisional diagnosis (Fig. 5.17). Because the film is swollen with water, interpretation of fine detail should wait until the film is dry. The film should remain in the fixer for at least 10 minutes to harden the gelatin and then be transferred to the wash tank.

The film should be washed in running water for half an hour.

Drying

The usual method of drying a small quantity of films is to take them out of the channel hangers, attach drying clips and hang them on a tensioned wire line in a dust-free place where there is a free air circulation. The films should not touch each other.

The effects of X-rays on living tissues are always harmful, but the practical results of such exposure depend on the amount and characteristics of the radiation and on the nature of the tissue irradiated.

In the early days of radiography, the pioneer workers did not at first realize that their new means of diagnosis was harmful or, if they did, they turned a blind eye to it and ignored the reddening of the skin which occurred around their nails. The early X-ray apparatus was crude and completely unshielded and the operators must have received massive doses of radiation. Those of the early workers who persisted in practising radiography died of cancer after terrible radiation injuries—which has justly entitled them to be called 'the X-ray martyrs'. It has been estimated that by 1922 about a hundred radiologists had died from radiation injury.

A number of veterinary surgeons are also known to have sustained X-ray injuries, but when one recalls the early ignorance of these dangers and the practical problems of restraining and handling uncooperative veterinary patients, this is hardly surprising. These risks are still present for the foolhardy and careless, but, provided they fully understand and adopt all necessary routine precautions, modern veterinary radiographers can reduce them to acceptable levels for themselves and their assistants.

The nature of radiation injury

X-rays produce changes within living cells when they are absorbed. There are a number of theories about the exact mechanism of the biological effect, but it can be broadly stated that the X-ray beam, when traversing a tissue, causes electrons to be ejected from the atomic lattice and leaves the atoms with a surplus positive electrical charge. The ionized cells within the tissue are then in a state of high chemical reactivity and the subsequent chemical reaction can initiate any one of three main biological effects.

1   *The Somatic Effect.* Radiation can produce immediate changes in the cell, although this damage may not become visible for some time, or may even be repaired and never appreciated. When damage is more extensive however, either through a single massive exposure or smaller repeated exposures, injury becomes apparent. Body cells are not equally sensitive to radiation, and healing after an injury also differs between cell types.

The most radiosensitive cells are those that are multiplying continuously, whereas the least sensitive are those that do not reproduce in the adult state. Thus the gonads, immature blood cells and the germinative layers of the skin and intestinal epithelium are most sensitive, while mature blood cells, muscle cells and connective tissue are relatively insensitive. Radiation of the lens of the eye can also cause damage and this may lead to cataract formation.

The developing fetus is particularly sensitive to radiation and young individuals are also at greater risk than adults to radiation injury because of their more rapidly reproducing cells. In radiotherapy this fact is employed to the patient's advantage in the use

Chapter 6

Radiation
Protection

of irradiation to destroy the rapidly multiplying cells of malignant tumours.

2 *The Carcinogenic Effect.* It is known that tissues which have been exposed to X-rays show a higher incidence of subsequent cancerous changes, although it may be many years before malignancies develop.

3 *The Genetic Effect.* Exposure of the gonads to radiation can produce both the somatic effect and the long-term genetic effect. The latter increases the mutation rate and, while causing no obvious harmful effects at the time, may produce inherited abnormalities in subsequent generations.

While these effects may result from exposure to single large doses of radiation, they can also be caused by relatively small amounts repeated over long periods.

The source of X-ray exposure

X-rays are produced at the anode of the X-ray tube only at the time of making an exposure. Persons adjacent to the apparatus may be exposed to such rays through any of the following means.

The tube head

Modern X-ray machines are designed to be as radiation-safe as possible. The X-ray tube is shielded with lead, except at the aperture where the beam emerges. Here filtration removes the unwanted 'soft rays' and the beam is then confined by a cone or diaphragm.

However, in this connection 'safe' is a relative term, particularly with regard to older machines. Therefore the tube head should never be held while in use. If there is any suspicion that the lead shielding is not effective one should consult a competent X-ray engineer or other expert. A simple way to check for oneself is to strap a piece of film (envelope wrapped or in a light-proof container) to the tube, make a number of exposures and then process the film. Any blackening of the emulsion will indicate that X-rays are penetrating the shielding. Similarly one should also check that the aluminium filters have not been removed from the aperture, thus permitting the emergence of useless, but potentially harmful, long wavelength X-rays.

The primary beam

The term *primary* or direct radiation refers to the emergent beam from the X-ray tube window. It should be collimated and filtered by aluminium. The primary beam poses the greatest risk of exposure to irradiation when undertaking diagnostic radiography because, unless a light beam diaphragm is used, it is not easy to estimate the exact position and extent of that beam, particularly if it is directed horizontally. It must be stressed that the primary beam is capable of penetrating protective clothing (lead aprons and gloves) and that *no person should be exposed to it, even if protected by this means.* In addition, it is not always remembered that the primary beam will penetrate unprotected table tops and can be a sometimes unappreciated hazard to the lower limbs of anyone holding a patient. Similarly, if the primary beam is directed at a thin wall or floor, persons on the other side of such a barrier may be at risk.

Secondary radiation (scatter)

This is emitted in all directions when the beam traverses the patient or reaches the X-ray table (Fig. 6.1). It is of lower intensity and less penetrating power than the primary beam and is absorbed by protective clothing. Because it travels in all directions some

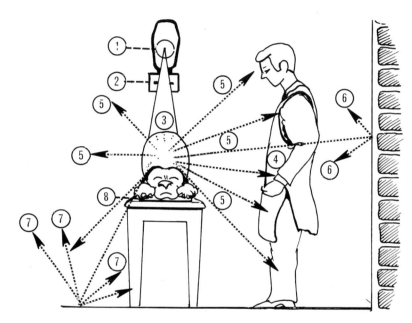

exposure to secondary radiation cannot be avoided by persons in the same room but the actual amount received is subject to the inverse square law (see p. 115) and rapidly decreases with distance. Provided, therefore, that strict precautions are adopted (see p. 106) this risk can be reduced to an acceptable one.

Fig. 6.1 The spread of scattered radiation:
1: Lead tube shield to prevent leakage radiation.
2: Beam collimator.
3: Primary beam.
4: Lead apron.
5: Scatter radiation from animal and table top.
6: Indirect scatter from wall.
7: Indirect scatter from floor.
8: Lead sheet in cassette.

Fluoroscopy (screening)

The dangers associated with the use of fluoroscopy have already been mentioned in Chapter 2, when the principles of the apparatus necessary for this procedure were described.

The main reason why fluoroscopy entails an increased risk of exposure to X-rays is the fact that the primary beam is activated for periods which are measured in minutes, rather than the fractions of a second necessary to expose a conventional radiograph. In addition, a principal veterinary indication for the use of fluoroscopy is the evaluation of alimentary function by observing the passage of a barium meal. Unfortunately the use of general anaesthesia or heavy sedation is likely to affect normal bowel activity, and so some restraint and positioning of the patient by assistants may be necessary. Obviously a combination of these two problems will greatly increase the risk, mentioned earlier, of exposure to secondary radiation and, unless great care is taken, to the primary beam.

Therefore fluoroscopic examinations should only be undertaken if the following requirements can be fulfilled:

1   Such an investigation is necessary in order to demonstrate a functional rather than a morphological abnormality in the patient.
2   Suitably constructed image intensification apparatus incorporating adequate protective devices (see p. 34) is available. Under no circumstances should one of the older X-ray machines (designed primarily for routine radiography but provided with simple fluoroscopy controls) be used in conjunction with hand-held fluoroscopes.
3   The examination is conducted by an experienced veterinary radiologist and all staff taking part are fully instructed in their duties, wear protective clothing and carry monitoring badges to record the amount of radiation received.

The maximum permissible dose

It is not possible to avoid some exposure to X-rays without discontinuing their use entirely, and the concept of the 'maximum permissible dose' has been introduced to denote an amount of irradiation which does not involve a greater risk to health than that encountered in other walks of life. The maximum permissible doses may be defined as levels of irradiation of an individual, or part of an individual, exposed in the course of his work, that are at present considered to constitute a safe threshold. Such doses should not be exceeded, and every effort should be made to keep the doses well below this level.

In order to make it possible to quantify the amount of radiation actually received certain terms have been introduced and are defined as follows:

1   *Absorbed Dose* is the quantity of energy imparted by ionizing radiations to matter per unit mass of the matter. The unit of absorbed dose is the *gray* (Gy). This replaces the previously used unit which was known as the *rad* (1 Gy = 100 rad).
2   *Dose Equivalent* is the quantity obtained by multiplying the absorbed dose in tissue by the quality factor so as to take account of the differing biological effectiveness of equal absorbed doses and other modifying factors. The unit of dose equivalent is the *sievert* (Sv) and this has superseded the rem which was previously employed for this purpose (1 Sv = 100 rem).
Note: At present the quality factor for X-rays is 1 and the product of the other modifying factors is also 1, and therefore the dose equivalent is numerically equal to the absorbed dose.

The actual amount of the maximum permissible dose is reviewed regularly by the responsible authorities and revised figures are issued from time to time. The amounts which apply at the time of writing are summarized in Table 6.1.

The maximum permissible dose is set at a much lower level for the general public because they will not be monitored and they are not trained to recognize and avoid accidental exposure. In

Table 6.1 Maximum permissible dose (in any calendar year).

	For persons at work aged 18 years or over (classified persons)	For trainees aged between 16 and 18 years	For any other persons
For the whole body	0.05 Sv (5 rem)	0.015 Sv (1.5 rem)	0.005 Sv (0.5 rem)
For individual organs and tissues	0.5 Sv (50 rem)	0.15 Sv (15 rem)	0.05 Sv (5 rem)
For the lens of the eye	0.15 Sv (1.5 rem)	0.05 Sv (5 rem)	0.03 Sv (3 rem)

In the case of women of reproductive capacity who are at work the dose to the abdomen may not exceed:

In any consecutive three months	0.013 Sv (1.3 rem)
If pregnant, during the period of pregnancy	0.01 Sv (1 rem)

A 'woman of reproductive capacity' is defined as 'any woman aged 16 years or over, except women who have been certified by a doctor that they are not of reproductive capacity'.

addition, on account of the large number of persons involved, the risk of genetic damage assumes far greater importance.

The actual amount of irradiation received by those engaged in radiography can be monitored. This is done by wearing small dosemeters which are sent regularly to an appropriate unit where they are processed and the dosage received calculated.

The permissible dose does not represent a large amount of direct radiation and such a dose can easily be exceeded if staff are exposed to the primary beam. On the other hand, *provided that the recommended precautions are observed* a large number of animals can be radiographed without anyone receiving a significant amount of irradiation.

PRECAUTIONARY MEASURES

Premises

The constructional factors to be considered in the selection of a particular part of a veterinary hospital for undertaking radiography are discussed on p. 120. The essential requirement is that X-ray examinations should be undertaken only in a clearly marked and suitable room in which there is no likelihood of the entry of unauthorized persons during the procedure or of the irradiation of nearby workers. Entry to the room should be restricted by notices, by displaying the international radiation symbol and by warning lights which are linked to the X-ray apparatus and are illuminated when exposures are being made (Fig. 6.2).

It is occasionally necessary to radiograph animals outside the designated area (e.g. at a farm or stable). In these circumstances portable warning signs forbidding access by unauthorized persons should be available and placed around the area in which radiography is being performed (Fig. 6.3). If it is necessary to use a horizontal beam it should always be directed towards a thick brick or similarly protective wall.

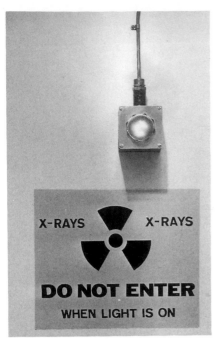

Fig. 6.2 Warning sign.

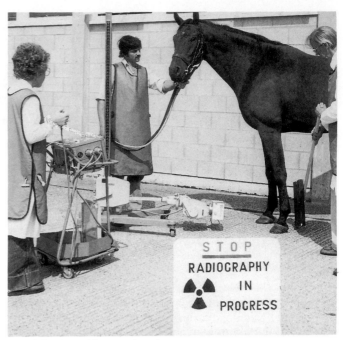

Fig. 6.3 Portable warning sign.

Equipment

New X-ray apparatus obtained from a reputable dealer or manufacturer will have been designed to comply with safety requirements.

Old and second-hand equipment should be inspected by a reliable X-ray engineer and may need modification before it can be safely used. As well as having poor shielding of the tube head, such machines can have had the aluminium filters removed or may lack remote control exposure buttons (which can be operated by means of a cable from a safe distance) or warning lights.

The fitting of a light beam diaphragm to any new or old X-ray machine facilitates visualization of the primary beam and contributes greatly to the safe use of such apparatus.

Protective clothing

Aprons

Aprons are designed to protect the body against scattered radiation and should be of a minimum of 0.25 mm lead equivalent for voltages up to 150 kV. They are usually made of plastic impregnated with lead and are reasonably hard wearing and easy to clean. The plastic and lead mixture may be manufactured as a single layer or as several thin layers. The latter is more flexible and easier to wear but inevitably more expensive.

The catalogues list many different styles and garments can be made to individual specification. The cheapest garments are the single-sided type which is strapped to the body. Although they are adequate, they are uncomfortable to wear for long periods. The double-sided form is easier to wear and provides better protection (Fig. 6.4).

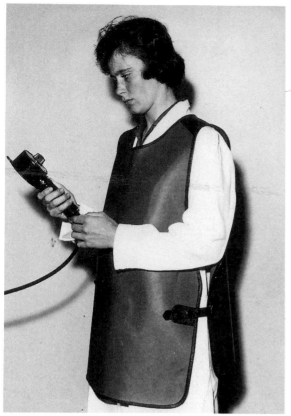
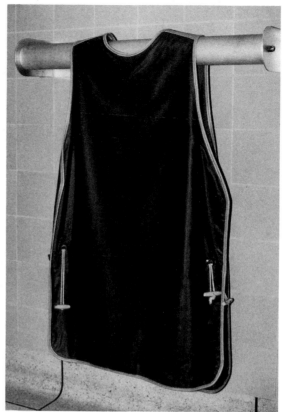

Fig. 6.4   **Fig. 6.5**

The aprons usually extend down to the thigh region, as their main purpose is to protect the chest and abdomen, but if a large amount of equine limb radiography is undertaken, longer aprons should be provided to protect the legs of assistants.

Gloves

There is a wide range of choice of types, sizes and lead equivalents, although for veterinary work, where the hands of those restraining the patient may have to be positioned fairly near the primary beam, the lead equivalent should not be less than 0.35 mm for voltages up to 150 kV.

Standard gloves made of lead rubber (Fig. 6.6) are available but are very easily damaged by fractious patients. They are therefore usually employed inside detachable leather covers but these are clumsy and awkward to use.

A number of devices are employed to permit better use of the hands during radiography (e.g. when injecting contrast media or restraining uncooperative animals). These include sheets or cuffs of lead rubber (Fig. 6.7), hand shields and mittens with open palms.

Care of protective clothing

Protective clothing is easily damaged by careless use or storage

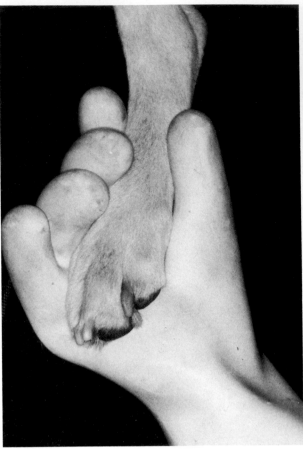

Fig. 6.6

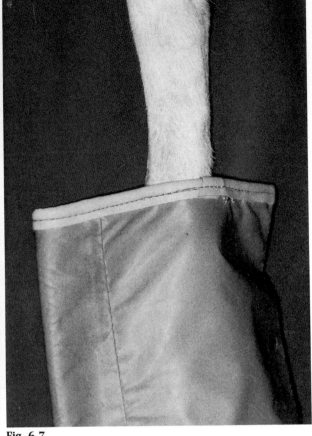

Fig. 6.7

and, since cracks in the material are not always obvious (e.g. when hidden by leather glove covers), this can be an unsuspected source of exposure to radiation.

Aprons should never be folded, as this will lead to cracking. When not in use they should be hung on stout hangers or rails not less than 3 cm in diameter (see Fig. 6.5).

As well as checking visually, all items of protective clothing should be subjected to a particularly thorough examination at least once a year. If there is any doubt concerning the completeness of the lead protection, it should be checked by placing a cassette under the article and making a fairly high exposure. If development of the film reveals any significant defects, the affected glove or apron should be discarded (Figs 6.8 and 6.9).

Each article should be individually marked and identified so that a record may be maintained indicating the dates of purchase and of subsequent examination for wear.

Lead screens

Mobile lead screens, which are usually provided with a lead glass window to permit observation of the patient, are a useful, but expensive, means of providing additional protection for staff within the X-ray room.

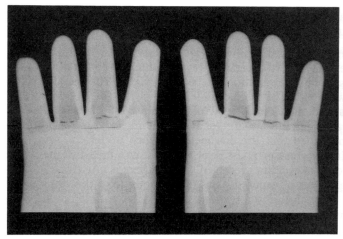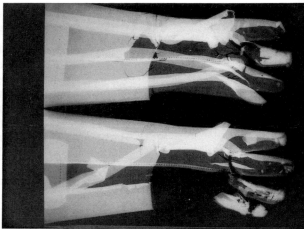

Dosemeters

The wearing of one of these monitoring devices is the only way of recording the actual amount of radiation received by those involved in radiography. They must be provided for all classified members of staff, but their provision also for those who take part in radiography less frequently can reassure radiation conscious members of staff and prevent any threat of subsequent litigation for imagined exposure to radiation.

Several types of monitoring badges are available:

1 *Film badges* are the simplest. They consist of a small piece of film in a lightproof envelope which is held in a plastic carrier that incorporates strips of tin and other metals which act as filters and thus determine the type of radiation. After possible exposure to X-rays the films are returned to a laboratory, where they are developed and any densities are measured. By comparing these figures with known standards, it is possible to calculate the amount of X-rays reaching the film and the equivalent dose received by the wearer.

These badges are accurate enough for most purposes but they cannot detect exposure levels of less than 0.2 mSv (20 mrem) and are subject to fogging by excessive heat, pressure or humidity.

2 *Thermoluminescent dosemeters* depend on the fact that when certain compounds (e.g. lithium fluoride and calcium fluoride) are heated they emit an amount of light directly proportional to the amount of radiation they have absorbed before heating. These compounds are available as fine crystals which are put into variously shaped small containers and worn by staff. In an appropriately equipped laboratory the amount of radiation received by the wearer of the dosemeter can be calculated with considerable accuracy. The advantages of this type of monitor are that measurements can be collected over a long period of time and that the size and shape of the device can be varied to suit particular purposes (they can be made very small for assessing any exposure to the fingers).

3 *Pocket ionization chambers* are more complex devices. They are approximately the size of a fountain pen and can be clipped to clothing. They are accurate and will give immediate readings but

Fig. 6.8 Cracking of the lead rubber at the usual site—the base of the fingers.

Fig. 6.9 Severe wear of the protective lead—not always appreciated if used under leather covering.

Radiographer

The title of 'radiographer' is used here for the person who will actually press the button and expose the film. Obviously he or she must understand something of the functioning of the apparatus, but the important point is that, whatever his status within the practice, he should have authority, for the purpose of conducting radiography, over all persons present in the X-ray room. He is then responsible for removing all unnecessary personnel and for checking that essential assistants are correctly positioned and protected, before making the exposure and releasing X-rays.

The general public

In order to reduce the amount of radiation to which staff are exposed, it is common practice to request members of the general public to assist in restraining their own animals during radiographic examinations. Provided that the owner concerned is capable of cooperating sensibly, this is fully justified, but care must be taken that the person involved gives this assistance only on a few occasions and that young people and pregnant women are never allowed to be present. The radiographer must check that such inexperienced assistants have been adequately instructed with regard to restraint of the patient and their own protection. He should be particularly vigilant to ensure that they are wearing suitable protective clothing and are correctly positioned in relation to the primary beam.

Safety routine before undertaking radiography

1   Decide if radiographic investigation is justified (owners often demand unnecessary X-ray examinations).
2   Decide whether, in the best interests of the patient and of the staff, the animal should be anaesthetized, sedated or manually restrained.
3   Remove all unnecessary persons from the room.
4   Check that all essential personnel are wearing protective clothing, and that they understand the part they are expected to play in the examination.
5   Check that the primary beam will be collimated to the required field and directed so that it will not irradiate people in adjacent rooms.
6   See that all assistants are positioned as far as possible from the primary beam and will not be exposed to it.
7   Press the button and make the exposure.

LEGAL LIABILITY

As the person responsible for potentially dangerous equipment, a veterinary surgeon has a moral obligation to ensure that it is used in such a way as to maintain the well being of his employees, the general public and their offspring. However, to an increasing degree, the use of X-ray equipment is being controlled and directed

by general and specific legislation. Obviously precise legal requirements will vary from country to country, but they will follow the
same general pattern.

Under English common law an employer has always been
required to provide a safe work place, safe plant and appliances
and a safe system of work and must exercise due care in the
appointment of employees in positions in which the safety of
others may depend upon their competence. An employer cannot
delegate these responsibilities. These requirements have now been
elaborated and made more specific by the Health and Safety at
Work etc. Act of 1974.

Since then, and following the recommendations of the International Commission on Radiological Protection and the issue of
the European Communities Directive of July 15 1980, on basic
safety standards in connection with ionizing radiation, the *Ionizing
Radiations Regulations 1985* have been drawn up and are now in
force. The issue of these regulations was accompanied by an
explanatory code of practice *The protection of persons against ionizing radiation arising from any work activity* which endeavours to
explain the implications of the new regulations for all potential
users of ionizing radiations and also contains a few specific ref-
erences to the employment of diagnostic radiography in veterinary
practice. It is the intention of the Health and Safety Executive to
issue a code of practice intended solely for veterinary radiography
some time in 1986, but a Consultative Document entitled *Draft
guidance notes for the protection of persons against ionizing radiations
arising from veterinary use,* on which the new code will be based,
has been available for some years. These publications are, or will
be, available from Her Majesty's Stationery Office and should be
studied by all those engaged in veterinary radiography.

The new regulations are inevitably somewhat legalistic and it
will require several years experience of their interpretation and
enforcement before it will be possible to say exactly how they will
apply to the very variable conditions under which radiography is
performed in veterinary practice.

The following notes are an attempt to summarize the main
requirements of the new legislation.

1   *Notification of the appropriate authority* (The Health and Safety
Executive) *of the intention to commence using apparatus capable of
producing ionizing radiations* (e.g. an X-ray machine) *in a veterinary
practice.* Such notification must be in writing and preferably using
a simple form which may be obtained from area offices of the
Health and Safety Executive.
2   *The assignment of ultimate responsibility within a practice for
radiological protection measures and the way in which these should be
put into effect.* The ultimate responsibility for radiological protection measures lies with the person or persons responsible for
the control of the veterinary practice or establishment, although
they may delegate the day to day supervision of such measures
by appointing a suitably experienced member of staff as Radiation
Protection Supervisor.

The principal must ensure that all members of staff liable to be
involved in radiographic procedures are adequately instructed

about the hazards they may meet and the precautions to be observed. He must also arrange for local rules (see p. 110) to be drawn up setting out clearly and precisely the procedures which are to be adopted for radiography.

3   *Definition of the area or areas in which radiography may be undertaken, and a means of preventing unauthorized access to such areas when exposures are being made.* The area selected must be one which can be clearly defined and described (e.g. a consulting room) and should be designated as either a 'controlled' or a 'supervised' area. The former term is used when a person working in the area might receive a dose of radiation exceeding three-tenths of the annual dose limit for adult workers, whereas if the estimated dose is likely to be less than this but still exceeds one-tenth of the annual dose limit, then the room should be a 'supervised area'. The particular designation may have to be decided upon after consultation with a Radiation Protection Adviser and is of significance in relation to the supervision of persons permitted to work in these areas.

The area selected must have a notice or sign forbidding entrance and these may only be removed or switched off when the X-ray apparatus has been disconnected from its source of power.

The regulations do however contain one important modification of the above requirements for veterinary purposes, but which may be implemented only when certain conditions can be fulfilled. These conditions are:

a   There is only one X-ray machine in the room and its beam is always directed vertically.

b   A collimating device ensures that the primary beam cannot come within 10 cm of the edge of the table.

c   The table is covered by 1 mm of lead over an area extending not less than 10 cm further in each direction than the largest area of the primary beam.

d   The apparatus operates at less than 100 kV.

e   The workload does not exceed 240 mAs in any one week.

The controlled area will then exist between the ceiling and the floor in a vertical direction and extending 1 metre out from each edge of the table.

This concession could obviously simplify the allocation of an area in which radiography may be undertaken but it will be invalidated if:

a   It is necessary to direct the primary beam horizontally (e.g. for demonstrating gas or fluid levels or for most equine examinations).

b   Anyone needs to place themselves or any part of their person within the controlled area while an exposure is being made. It will therefore be necessary to anaesthetize all patients for radiography.

c   There is a possibility of the stated workload being exceeded during any *one* week in the year (240 mAs is very roughly equivalent to some 40 small animal exposures—and probably represents a larger number of examinations when fast films and screens are employed).

4   *The selection of staff who are liable to be exposed to ionizing*

radiations in the course of their duties and, after estimation of the amount of radiation to which they may be subjected, their classification or organization under an appropriate scheme of work. The regulations require that any person who, in the course of his work, might be exposed to radiation which could exceed three-tenths of any of the dose limits, should be designated as a 'classified person' and made subject to further controls. No person under 18 years of age or any pregnant woman may be so classified. In addition those appointed must first be certified fit for the work by an approved doctor and the amount of radiation they receive must be regularly monitored.

It is very unlikely that those taking part in radiography in veterinary practice will be exposed to the amount of radiation mentioned above unless they are required to position themselves close to the primary beam for the restraint of a large number of conscious patients. Provided, therefore, that the likely radiographic workload has been estimated and the risk to staff checked, the regulations require that those who do not need to be classified should be organized under a written scheme of work as suggested on p. 110.

5 *The provision of suitable and safe apparatus.* All new X-ray apparatus is required to satisfy extremely high standards of safety in use. In addition the installer of such equipment must critically review the way in which this has been done and must supply the operator with adequate information concerning the proper use of the apparatus.

Second-hand apparatus should always be checked by an experienced X-ray engineer and rejected if it does not meet the necessary standards of safety in use.

6 *The obtaining, when in doubt, of expert advice on all aspects of safety precautions.* The regulations require that, when there is any doubt concerning the adequacy of the safety precautions, a Radiation Protection Adviser (who may be an individual or an organization specializing in such work) should be appointed. This appointment may be for a single consultation or on an ongoing basis. Only suitably qualified and experienced physicists or other specialists are acceptable for this purpose and their names must be submitted to the Health and Safety Executive for approval, before appointment.

It is suggested that such an adviser should be selected from one of the following sources:

a Radiation Protection Advisers in universities or colleges of technology.
b Hospital physicists.
c The National Radiological Protection Board or the Northern Ireland Radiation Protection Service.
d Suitably experienced holders of the Diploma in Veterinary Radiology.

At the time of writing it is likely that the experts classified under (a), (b) and (c) above will lack experience of the problems peculiar to the practice of veterinary radiography and that those coming under (d) will not possess the necessary radiation investigative and monitoring apparatus. It is to be hoped that these groups will share their expertise and that, within a few years, a comprehensive advisory service will be available.

Specimen local rules

These are copied from those in the *Draft Guidance Notes for the Protection of Persons Against Ionising Radiations arising from Veterinary Use* and are reproduced with the permission of the Controller of Her Majesty's Stationery Office.

1   These local rules are issued by the principal and are intended to ensure that the X-ray set is used safely and in accordance with the requirements of the Ionising Radiations Regulations 1985 and the associated approved code of practice. They are consistent with the 'Guidance Notes for the Protection of Persons exposed to Ionising Radiations arising from Veterinary Use'. They must be read and understood by all staff.

2   *Radiation protection adviser*
The principal has appointed the National Radiological Protection Board of 155 Hardgate Road, Glasgow as radiation protection adviser.

3   *Radiation protection supervisor*
The principal has appointed John Doe, radiation protection supervisor (RPS). He shall administer the local rules, the requirements of the regulations and approved code and the recommendations of the 'guidance notes' and shall report to the principal.

4   *Controlled area*
The X-ray room is designated as a controlled area. Staff who are not 'classified persons' may remain in this room during radiography only in accordance with the 'scheme of work' described below.

5   *Classified persons*
The following members of staff are designated as classified persons and may take part routinely in radiography: John Doe, Richard Roe are under medical supervision and wear personal dosemeters. They must read and understand the relevant sections of the 'guidance notes'. Each classified person must bear in mind that it is his duty to protect himself and others from the hazards associated with radiography.

6   *Scheme of work*
Staff who are not classified persons may not take part routinely in radiography. Occasional participation, on not more than five occasions per month, must be authorised on each occasion by the RPS, who shall decide whether personal dosemeters should be worn.

7   *X-ray room*
Radiography shall be carried out, normally, in the room marked with the warning sign which incorporates the trefoil radiation symbol. During radiography, the 'no entry' sign shall be hung on the door of the X-ray room. Exceptionally, radiography may be carried out elsewhere, but only with the express permission of the RPS who shall specify the conditions of use.

8   *X-ray set*
The X-ray set may not be modified so as to alter its performance or shielding except with the express permission of the RPS. Any malfunction shall be reported immediately to him.

9   *Radiography procedures*
John Doe and Richard Roe are appointed 'radiographers' and shall supervise radiographic procedures; in that capacity they shall have authority over all persons present at an examination and shall exclude all unauthorised and unessential persons. The examination shall be carried out in accordance with Chapter 7 of the 'guidance notes'. (A notice should be posted in the X-ray room detailing radiographic procedures as recommended in 7.1.4. The correct sequence of actions should be listed,

for example: Immobilise the animal. Position the animal and cassette. Select exposure factors and beam size. Don protective apron and stand as far as practicable from the path of the useful beam. Warn persons present of imminent exposure and then take the radiograph. Switch off X-ray set so as to prevent unintentional exposure. Any special points, such as a restriction on beam direction specified by the radiation protection adviser, should also be included in the notice.)

10 *Personal dosemeters*

Persons issued with personal dosemeters must wear them at all times during work and report damage or loss of the badges to the RPS who shall replace them. When not in use, dosemeters must be kept outside the X-ray room, dry and away from heaters.

11 *Protective clothing*

All persons authorised to be present during radiography must wear protective aprons which must be replaced on the rail after use. Persons who are asked by the radiographer to hold animals must cover their hands and forearms with protective drapes.

12 *Visitors*

No visitors shall be allowed to remain in the X-ray room or radiography area during radiography except for owners of animals when their assistance is needed for restraining the animal. They shall be given clear instructions on their role.

Authors' note

The inclusion of 'Classified persons' in the above suggests that the rules are intended for a particularly busy X-ray unit where there is a possibility of staff receiving more than three-tenths of the maximum permissible dose. This is unlikely to occur in general practice, particularly if radiography is used responsibly, and in these circumstances paragraph 5 might be omitted and paragraph 6 expanded to provide more information concerning how and when staff might take part in radiographic examinations.

Risks to the patient

This chapter has been concerned with the dangers of irradiation as they affect people, rather than animals. This has been done because, putting on one side the very emotive arguments concerning the relative importance of animals and humans, the veterinary surgeon and his assistants are likely to be involved in many more radiographic examinations than one individual animal and the risk to the patient may, in general, be discounted. However, bearing in mind the susceptibility of the fetus and the incompletely understood genetic effects of radiation, it is advisable to avoid excessive and unnecessary radiography of pregnant females and of the testicular region of males likely to be used for breeding (if necessary the testicles can be protected with a lead shield).

Chapter 7

The Estimation of Exposure

The aim of the radiographer must always be to select those exposure factors, which, in conjunction with the radiographic apparatus and technique employed, will produce a radiograph showing optimum visualization of the part under examination. While tables of suitable exposures are available and are included in Appendix 2, there are so many variable factors involved that the first radiographs will always involve a certain amount of trial and error. The radiographer must, therefore, be aware of all these causes of variation in order that he can correct errors in the radiographs produced and, so that, once an acceptable film is obtained, he may maintain a consistent standard in films of other patients.

By keeping a record of the size of the patient (weight or thickness of tissue) and all the exposure factors employed, the radiographer can then make up his own exposure chart, based on the results of his own work on his own machine and on his own concept of what constitutes a good diagnostic radiograph.

This chapter is concerned with the many different factors which affect exposure estimation and with the re-calculations which have to be made when a factor is altered, such as the employment of a different focal–film distance or when dealing with increased tissue thickness.

Standardization and simplification by reducing the number of variable factors will be considered at the end of this chapter.

THE FACTORS INVOLVED IN AN X-RAY EXPOSURE

X-ray machine

Make and type
Input voltage
Kilovoltage
Milliamperage
Time
Focal–film distance
Collimation of X-ray beam

Patient

Thickness of part
Nature of part
Pathological changes within part
Movement
Dressing and casts

Cassette

Film type and speed
Intensifying screen factor
Grid factor

Dark room

Correct and incorrect development

Radiograph

Individual preference

All these factors have an effect on the finished film, and if any one factor is altered without compensation, there will be a difference in the image produced.

Make and type of X-ray apparatus

Exposure factors which have proved satisfactory for one particular X-ray machine should be suitable for use with other machines of the same make, but this is not always true as individual variation does occur. Similarly factors which apply to one type of portable machine will provide a rough guide for the use of other portable apparatus. On the other hand, readings used on the smaller half-wave rectified apparatus will not be applicable to full wave or constant potential machines.

Input voltage

The significance of this factor is dealt with in Chapter 2. Failure to correct fluctuations will result in a very variable output negating all other efforts at standardization of exposure.

Kilovoltage

The kilovoltage control regulates the penetrating power of the X-ray beam because the tension applied to the ends of the tube is proportional to the 'hardness' of the radiation produced.

The initial selection of kilovoltage for a given part must be made empirically and repeated until a film is obtained showing detail within the densest portions (e.g. bone), without over-penetration and obliteration of the more radiotranslucent areas. The use of too high kilovoltage will result in a 'flat' film which lacks contrast.

Having obtained a satisfactory radiograph, the kilovoltage can be varied for other patients in relation to the thickness of the part. Various rule-of-thumb calculations have been advised for making such alterations but none are precise. As a rough guide, the author would suggest adjusting by 1.5 kV for each centimetre of soft tissue difference. When dealing with the chest or with a predominantly bony area the variation should be nearer 1 kV and 2 kV per centimetre of thickness respectively.

There are also circumstances, other than an increase in tissue thickness, in which it may be helpful to use higher kilovoltage values.

The first of these is encountered when radiographing structures showing marked variation in radiodensity (e.g. dorsoventral projections of the chest). In these circumstances it can be helpful to deliberately over-penetrate the area using high kilovoltage, but to compensate for this by reducing the milliamperage-seconds. This should result in a more uniform visualization of both the dense and the translucent portions of the film.

Another reason for raising the kilovoltage above the optimum is to reduce the exposure time when using apparatus of low milliamperage output. The relation between kV and mA-s is a complicated one but works out roughly as follows—an increase of 10 kV will permit decreasing the mA-s (usually the time) by 50 per cent. The converse (a decrease of 10 kV needs to be compensated by a 50 per cent increase in the mA-s values) is also approximately true.

Milliampere-seconds

Because of their close relationship the significance of milli-amperage and time are best considered together.

Most X-ray apparatus permits the milliamperage to be adjusted but it is advisable to use the portable machines at their maximum setting (15 or 20 mA) in order to keep the exposure time as low as possible.

The duration of an exposure should be as short as possible for conscious animals, but even when anaesthetized, involuntary movement can blur a film and make it diagnostically useless.

Ideally, exposures should not exceed 0.1 second, because of the constant hazard of movement. This is not always possible when using low output X-ray apparatus but, if fast (rare-earth) screens and films are available, it should be practicable when X-raying most areas of small and medium-sized dogs.

Patient thickness and exposure time

When using small apparatus in which the kilovoltage is also limited, exposure differences in relation to body thickness must usually be made by varying the time (mA will already be at the maximum value). Obviously, the penetrating power of the maximum kV can traverse only a certain volume of tissue before becoming completely absorbed. Any increase in exposure time after this stage has been reached will be useless (and will have also resulted in an exposure time that is too long to be practicable for veterinary purposes).

Calculations For each centimetre of tissue added (or subtracted) raise (or lower) the mA-s by 25 per cent.

With small portable units, only the exposure time need be varied. This does *not* mean that a patient which is 3 cm thicker requires 75 per cent more time, but

$$\frac{5}{4} \times \frac{5}{4} \times \frac{5}{4} = 1.95 \text{ (approximately 100 per cent increase)}$$

Table 7.1 gives the percentage of exposure time (or mA-s) which should be added (or subtracted) for increases or decreases of tissue thickness.

Table 7.1

cm	Percentage
1	25
2	50
3	100
4	150
5	200

Focal–film distance

The distance between the focal spot of the tube and the film is an important exposure value. Whenever possible it should be kept as a constant.

X-rays obey the laws of light in that they diverge from a point source. The intensity of the beam varies inversely according to the square of the distance (the *inverse square law*) (Fig. 7.1).

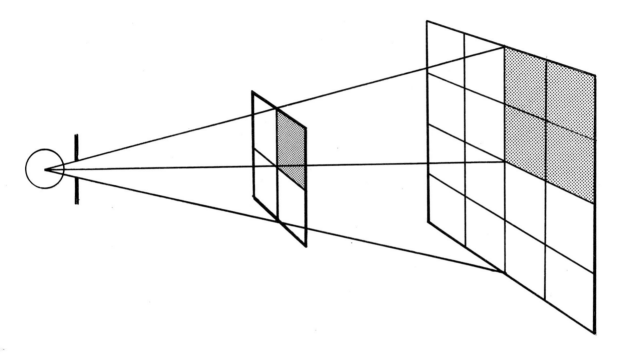

When a different distance is used, the adjustment is calculated thus:

$$\text{old mA-s} \times \frac{\text{new distance}^2}{\text{old distance}^2} = \text{new mA-s}$$

e.g.

$$10 \text{ mA-s} \times \frac{150^2 \text{ cm}}{75^2 \text{ cm}} = \frac{40}{1} = 40 \text{ mA-s}$$

Fig. 7.1 The inverse square law. The intensity of the beam falling on a given area is reduced to one quarter by doubling the distance from the point source.

Figure 7.2 shows the amount by which an mA-s factor suitable for a 75 cm focal–film distance must be multiplied to adjust for a change in distance.

With small apparatus a focal–film distance of 75 cm is usual, but a small amount of geometrical distortion must be accepted. If more powerful apparatus is available, 1 metre is preferred.

When the tube is directed horizontally, a measuring tape or stick should be used, so that the focal–film distance is always correct. This is especially important where both limbs are being taken for comparison.

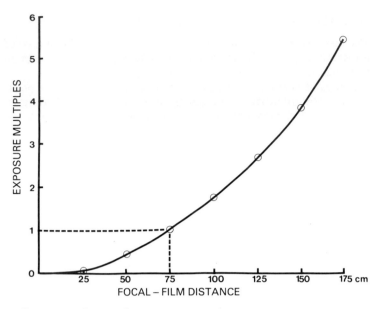

Fig. 7.2

Collimation of X-ray beam

The use of cones or other means of limiting the field of radiation is an essential means of protection and also a valuable method of reducing scatter. However, this also reduces the amount of blackening of the radiograph and when a particularly narrow cone is employed some increase in the exposure factors will be necessary to compensate for this.

The thickness and nature of the part and associated pathological changes

While, as already indicated, exposure factors are related to the thickness of the part being examined, the nature of the tissue and the presence or absence of any pathological changes within it, also have to be considered. Thus a given thickness of tissue may contain a high proportion of air (the chest), soft tissue (the abdomen) or bone (the equine limb), and each of these circumstances will require an increase in the amount of radiation (mA-s) or in its penetrating power (kV), or in both, if the part is to be correctly visualized. Similarly increased exposure factors will be necessary for the chest or abdomen if they contain appreciable amounts of fluid. On the other hand, loss of bone calcium in a patient will result in overexposure of the radiograph if not compensated for.

An experienced operator can often predict and compensate for these effects, but the first film of an examination is always experimental and may need to be repeated. The patient should never be sent away until the films have been processed and examined.

Movement

Movement of the conscious patient leading to blurring of the radiograph must always be a problem in veterinary radiography.

This can be minimized only by anaesthetization, sedation or other restraint of the patient and by employing the minimum practicable exposure time. Brief exposures require increased milliamperage but this is not possible with portable X-ray units and it may be necessary to attempt to compensate for this defect by employing increased kilovoltage, fast films and screens, or even by reducing the focal–film distance (a combination of all these modifications is likely to result in significant impairment of the radiographic image).

Dressings and casts

Wherever possible these should be removed. Wood and fabric need only a slight increase in exposure. Soft metals such as aluminium need about 5 kV more but steel splints are completely radio-opaque to the output of small sets. Dry plaster of paris needs twice the usual exposure. Wet casts need four times the exposure.

Films and intensifying screens

The significance of using different types of film has been discussed in Chapter 4. Briefly, the use of screen film in combination with intensifying screens permits the use of much lower exposure factors than when direct exposure film is employed. However, different types both of film and screen vary with regard to their speed. It is preferable therefore to always use the same film-screen combination, but should it be necessary to vary either, a compensatory adjustment of the exposure factors will have to be made.

It is worth pointing out that if ultra-fast films are used with high speed screens, or standard film with rare-earth screens, overexposure is likely to occur when radiographing the lower limbs of cats and small dogs (particularly if the timer does not go below 0.1 second).

Grids

The use of a grid will always involve an increase in exposure (usually the mA-s is increased by two to three times).

Processing

A precise and identical processing technique must be maintained if consistent radiographs are to be obtained. Underdevelopment (which may be due to development at too low a temperature or for too short a time, or to the use of exhausted developing solution) is a very common fault and will produce a film that appears to be 'underexposed' and shows poor contrast and a grey background. The opposite fault (overdevelopment) is of less significance but gross overdevelopment will produce a dark somewhat 'overexposed' film in which there is some blurring of detail as a result of fogging.

Individual preference

While it must be the aim of the radiographer to so select the exposure factors that all the radiographs are consistent in appearance, it is a matter of personal preference whether these are light or dark.

THE STANDARDIZATION OF EXPOSURE FACTORS

The above catalogue of factors has been listed in order to emphasize the large number of variables which can be involved in the estimation of radiographic exposure. If factors are to be selected logically and not on a 'trial and error' basis, it is advisable to adopt a definite routine on first undertaking the use of radiography or on obtaining new apparatus. This will involve:

1   *The standardization of as many factors as possible.*
   (*a*)   Check and correct any variations in the input voltage.
   (*b*)   Make sure that the film is placed at the same distance from the anode for all exposures. This is not easy to achieve when directing the beam in the oblique or horizontal plane.
   (*c*)   Use the same brand of processing chemicals consistently and check frequently that the solutions are maintained in a fresh condition and at the same temperature.

2   *The assessment and recording of optimum values for the adjustable factors* (*kilovoltage, milliamperage and time*). Suggested values may be obtained in the first place from published lists of exposure factors for similar machines (see pp. 355–366), but experience may show that it is necessary to adjust the published figures by a constant factor, to allow for slight variations in the machine or for the particular conditions under which radiography is undertaken.

Alternatively the radiographer may make a number of test exposures on an animal or carcase and then judge for himself the most successful results. It will economize, both in time and cost, if a series of different exposures of a part are made on portions of the same film after having protected the rest of the film with lead or other radio-opaque material. In making such trial exposures it is best to keep first the kV, and then the mA-s, constant and to use 3 or 4 settings of the other control—these representing a range of the figures at which the set is likely to be employed.

Once the most suitable exposure factors for the demonstration of particular areas (e.g. the skull, spine, distal limb, chest and abdomen of the dog, and the lower limb of the horse) have been assessed, these should be recorded in relation to the size of the patient (ideally by measuring the thickness of the part accurately) and made available when radiographing the same area in other animals. Adjustment can be made for animals of other sizes, bearing in mind the advice given earlier under kilovoltage and milliampere-seconds.

Where large X-ray machines giving a wide range of kV and mA settings are available, it is possible to produce exposure charts in which only one factor (either the kV or the mA-s) needs to be adjusted in relation to the exact depth of the part being examined. For a more detailed exposition of this technique the reader is referred to Morgan and Silverman (1982).

Once experience has been gained in selecting kV and mA-s settings under the conditions described above, it will be possible to adapt these to allow for other variations which are likely to include:

1 The use of a grid.
2 Changes in tissue density associated with pathological change.
3 The introduction of other types of film or intensifying screens, in order to extend the range of examinations undertaken.

Reference

Morgan, J. P. and Silverman, S. (1982) *Techniques of Veterinary Radiography*, 3rd ed. Davis, Calif.: Veterinary Radiology Associates.

APPARATUS

X-ray machines

The various types of X-ray apparatus available have been described in Chapter 2. Most machines have been manufactured for human use and, before purchasing a particular set, it is important to check that it will be suitable for the veterinary purpose for which it will be employed. Suitability will depend very largely on the output of the apparatus (very low in the case of dental machines) and on its manœuvrability (particularly important for equine work).

Second-hand X-ray apparatus

Some saving can be achieved by purchasing second-hand X-ray apparatus, usually either as redundant equipment from a hospital or through an agency dealing with such machines. However, purchase of intricate apparatus by the inexperienced must always be something of a gamble and could result in one obtaining equipment which was unsafe electrically or radiologically and was a hazard in use. Therefore, unless obtained from a reliable source, it is essential to have such apparatus checked by a suitably trained expert (e.g. an X-ray service engineer) to ensure that it is safe to use and that it fulfils all the requirements of the Ionizing Radiation Regulations 1985.

The following points should also be borne in mind when contemplating obtaining second-hand X-ray machines.

Many of the older units are no longer manufactured, and there can be difficulty in obtaining spare parts or servicing facilities.

Some X-ray apparatus has been devised solely for specialized human examinations (e.g. dental and skull units, fluoroscopic apparatus) and may not be suitable for general veterinary purposes.

In general, the larger and more intricate fixed apparatus is likely to be relatively cheaper than the popular portable and mobile equipment. However, it will require considerable space and the cost of transportation, installation and maintenance is likely to be much higher.

ACCESSORY APPARATUS

Essential items such as films, cassettes, grids and processing equipment have already been described in Chapters 4 and 5. There are, however, a number of other pieces of equipment which can be of assistance in the X-ray room.

Positioning equipment

The table
The most important requirement of any table used for veterinary radiography is rigidity, although it should not be fixed to the floor. Usually the table employed for clinical examinations serves both purposes. It is essential to line the under surface with lead to

absorb any portion of the primary beam which extends beyond the cassette. It can also be helpful to have suitable fittings for a compression band attached to the table.

Such tables usually have a smooth cleanable top which has the disadvantage that, when positioning a wriggling animal, the cassette tends to slide all over the table. This can be discouraged by purchasing a small rubber bathroom mat, preferably with a rough surface. The cassette and animal are placed on this and positioning is made easier.

Cassette stands

It is sometimes necessary to direct the primary beam horizontally (although the practice should be restricted as much as possible for reasons of safety) and film cassettes then have to be supported in a vertical position.

The practice of holding a cassette in the gloved hand cannot be justified. Gloves are only intended to protect against scattered radiation, not the primary beam, and cassettes should always be held in a suitable holder. Enthusiastic handymen will find some scope for devising these holders, as no single one will answer every need.

Below and overleaf are illustrated a few designs employed by the authors. No claim is made for their originality or that they cannot be improved.

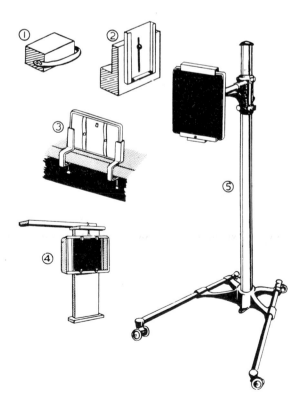

Fig. 8.1
1   A simple hardwood block with the cassette held vertically by a piece of rubber from an old tyre.
2   A more versatile holder made from 16 gauge aluminium sheet. It is bolted with a thumb-screw to another stout piece of metal which is screwed to a wooden block for stability. A vertical slit in the back of the holder enables the height to be raised. The angle of the cassette is also adjustable.
3   Two opposing metal channels, which grip the sides of the cassette, are mounted on 'G' clamps which fit on the edge of the table. Any size of cassette can be accommodated.
4   This is a cassette stand for the radiography of the legs of large animals. A simple wooden frame holds an 18 × 24 cm cassette which slides up and down a central wooden upright. A length of chain attached to the top of the cassette frame passes through a hole in the top of the stand and is hooked at the back at the appropriate height. A handle is fitted to the top to keep the assistant's gloved hand away from the beam.
5   A mobile cassette holder which is made from an old X-ray tube-column. It can be wound up to a height of 1.5 metres.

Fig. 8.6   Commercially available sandbags.

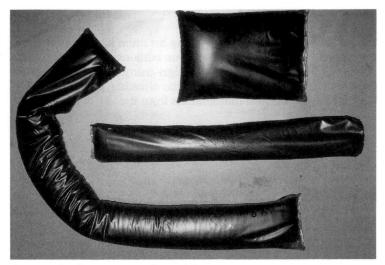

Accessories for equine radiography

Many of the cassette stands illustrated on p. 123 can be employed for large, as well as small animal examinations.

Fig. 8.7 illustrates a number of devices which are likely to be required when undertaking radiography of the feet and legs of horses. All can be constructed from wood by a carpenter.

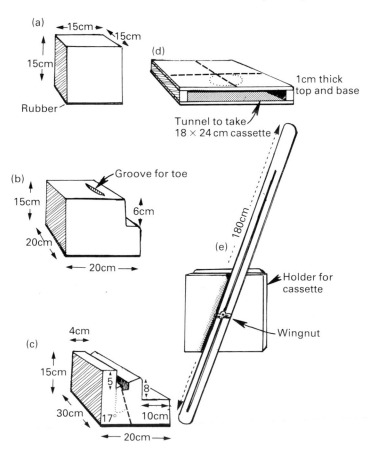

Fig. 8.7
- (a) A block useful for raising the foot above ground level
- (b) Pedal block
- (c) Navicular block
- (d) A strongly constructed cassette tunnel suitable for placing under a horse's foot.
- (e) The cassette holder already described on p. 124.

Fig. 8.8

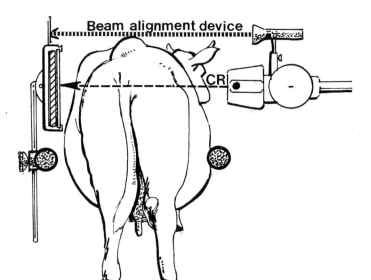

When high-power apparatus is available and radiography of the thorax, abdomen, spine or pelvis of large animals is attempted, the cassette is likely to be hidden from the radiographer and some means of centring the primary beam on the cassette and grid is essential. When radiographing the standing animal simple devices may be improvised to direct the beam at the cassette (e.g. Fig. 8.8), but where high ratio grids are also being used very precise alignment is essential and very sophisticated equipment (see Fig. 2.14, p. 32) is required.

If the vertical beam is employed to radiograph the anaesthetized animal difficulty will be encountered in positioning the cassette beneath the heavy mass of tissue. In these circumstances a strongly constructed cassette tunnel which also incorporates a centring device is helpful and is illustrated in Fig. 8.9.

MISCELLANEOUS EQUIPMENT

Masking the film

A considerable saving of film is effected, especially when radiographing the distal extremities, if the two projections of the limb are made on one film. Cassettes and film holders are usually marked on their front face, into quadrants. This enables half a film to be covered by a sheet of lead or lead-rubber while the other half is being exposed. The lead is transferred to the other half for the second exposure. Make sure that the lead does not cover the centre line twice or an ugly white line will appear on the radiograph between the two exposures.

Identification of the film

Opaque letters and numbers of different types can be purchased for placing on the cassette prior to exposure to record such relevant information as *Right* or *Left*, *Lateral* or *Medial*, etc. (Fig. 8.10).

Fig. 8.12   Ilford Viewing Lantern, Type 7.

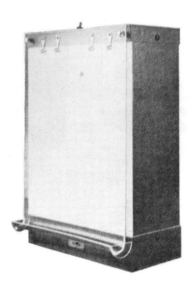

Protection equipment

Protection is such an important subject that a chapter has been devoted to it. The relevant equipment has been discussed on pp. 100–102.

Domiciliary visits

If it is likely that X-ray machines will be taken out on domiciliary visits, portable warning signs (see p. 100) should be available so that the area in which radiography is being undertaken can be clearly designated.

Always check that a suitable power outlet is available before undertaking such a visit.

STAFF

If the radiographic unit is to be used efficiently it is important that one member of the professional staff should assume responsibility for the safe use of these facilities and should spend time becoming proficient both in the technique of radiography and in the art of interpreting radiographs.

Provided that such experienced and interested supervision is available, it is possible to delegate responsibility for all dark room work and for some routine radiography to suitably trained assistants. Lay staff should not, however, be expected to assume complete responsibility for radiography. This is stressed, both because the veterinary surgeon in charge can never delegate his responsibility for the safe use of X-ray apparatus, and because good radiographic technique requires an understanding of the anatomy and likely pathology of the part being radiographed.

MINIMUM EQUIPMENT REQUIRED

The authors felt that it might be useful to conclude this chapter by giving a list of what, in addition to the X-ray machine, they consider to be the minimum requirements for the satisfactory establishment of a veterinary radiographic unit, and this is listed below. Additional equipment (e.g. a grid, other sized cassettes and frames) may be added as required.

Essential accessory equipment

Cassettes should be of robust construction—
  One 30 × 40 cm
  One 18 × 24 cm
Intensifying screens—several types are available; (rare-earth screens are more expensive, but have many advantages)
  One pair 30 × 40 cm
  One pair 18 × 24 cm
Lead-rubber strips for masking cassettes
Lead R and L letters.

Positioning Equipment
  Sandbags
  Foam rubber or other softpads
  Troughs
  Cassette holders, etc.
  A means of measuring the focal–film distance.

Dark Room Equipment (apart from fixtures)
  Processing dishes and heating plate
  or
  Processing tanks and immersion heater
  or
  A small processing unit
Processing frames (channel type)
  Two 30 × 40 cm
  Two 18 × 24 cm
  One pair of wall brackets
  One dozen drying clips
  Thermometer
  Clockwork film timer
  Wall safe-light and suitable filter (e.g. 'Wratten' 6B)
  Viewing box with protective wet film attachment

Protective Clothing
  Three double-sided protective aprons (minimum lead equivalent 0.25 mm)
  Two pairs protective gloves or hand shields (minimum lead equivalent 0.35 mm)

Expendable Material
  Films
    One box 50 folder wrapped 30 × 40 cm screen films
    One box 50 folder wrapped 18 × 24 cm screen films

The object of positioning for radiography is the devising of the most suitable postures in which the patient may be placed to facilitate:

1   The welfare of the patient.
2   The restraint and immobilization of the patient.
3   The most accurate reproduction of the part under examination in the radiograph produced.
4   The least risk of exposing those assisting with the examination to radiation.

The positioning suggested in the following pages has been developed and modified in the light of the experience of the authors and of their colleagues at the Cambridge University School of Veterinary Medicine, and has proved satisfactory in meeting the above requirements. However, it is not suggested that the techniques advocated are the only ones suitable for the particular radiological examination required, or that they cannot be improved upon.

Nomenclature

In the previous edition of this book the authors drew attention to the revised positional terminology which had been adopted by veterinary anatomists and which could affect the nomenclature used to describe the projections employed in veterinary radiography. At the time it was decided not to incorporate the new terminology into *Principles of Veterinary Radiography* until the revised anatomical terms were more widely used.

Since then, an American committee of veterinary radiologists and anatomists have published a report (Smallwood *et al,* 1985) in which they advocate the use of a new standardized terminology for veterinary radiographic projections. This system is based on the revised anatomical nomenclature and exactly defines the position and direction of the X-ray beam used for particular projections.

The new nomenclature is gaining acceptance and being increasingly used for scientific papers. It has, therefore, been introduced throughout the second half of this book, but the older, more familiar, terms have also been retained, since it is likely that they will continue to be used for some time to come.

The revised system is based on two simple rules:

1   Radiographic projections should be described using only accepted veterinary anatomical directional terms or their abbreviations. There are 14 of these terms:

Left (Le)	Medial (M)
Right (Rt)	Lateral (L)
Dorsal (D)	Proximal (Pr)
Ventral (V)	Distal (Di)
Cranial (Cr)	Palmar (Pa)
Caudal (Cd)	Plantar (Pl)
Rostral (R)	Oblique (O)

and their anatomical location is indicated in Fig. 9.1.
2   Using the above terms, radiographic projections should be described by the direction that the central ray of the primary beam

Chapter 9

General Principles

described in Part 2 of the book could be undertaken satisfactorily without the use of chemical restraint. In view of the availability of improved anaesthetic drugs and techniques, the considerably increased use of radiography in veterinary investigations and the greater awareness of the associated risks, that advice is now modified and, while general anaesthesia is not advocated as a routine for all examinations, its use is advised for a much larger number of the projections described. The decision to employ, or not to employ, such restraint can only be taken by the veterinarian concerned in the light of his knowledge of the full circumstances of a particular case—the dog's temperament and physical condition, the assistance available, the choice of anaesthetics and sedatives, and his own experience and skill in administering them. However, the principal arguments to be considered are described below.

General anaesthesia

General anaesthesia does provide the ideal conditions for positioning the patient (although the complete relaxation produced may have to be corrected by additional cushioning). It obviates the need for anyone to hold the patient during an exposure and thus reduces the radiation hazard to staff. In addition, the improved control of movement prevents unsatisfactory or wasted films due to blurring. Against this, the adoption of general anaesthesia solely for radiography is time-consuming, and may subject the patient to unnecessary risk. It is seldom practicable for large-animal examinations and may not be necessary for some routine small animal radiography. One must also bear in mind that it is dangerous to employ ether or other inflammable anaesthetics in close proximity to X-ray or other electrical apparatus.

In a few instances it may be possible to delay radiography until the patient is anaesthetized for operation and to take the necessary radiographs immediately prior to its admission to the operating theatre, thus avoiding the necessity for anaesthetizing the animal twice.

Sedation

Sedation also involves a delay before the patient can be radiographed. It restricts movement and facilitates restraint, but unless the patient is firmly supported and tied in position, some manual restraint may still be required.

Radiography of the conscious patient

Radiography of the conscious patient may be necessary with sick and shocked patients and for those suffering from severe respiratory disease thoracic radiography may be necessary before anaesthetization can be contemplated. However, it is more likely to result in spoilt films, and it must be very strictly organized and supervised if the risk of exposure to radiation is to be kept to a minimum (see Chapter 6).

Preparation of the patient

Preparation of the patient by means of general anaesthesia or sedation has just been discussed.

The other main need for preparation of the patient is to prevent the formation of confusing shadows on the radiograph due to such causes as faeces or gas in bowel, or external agents—dirt or harness. The former problem will be discussed further when dealing with radiography of the abdomen and contrast media techniques (Chapters 11 and 13). There are, however, several external causes of extraneous radiographic shadows which have to be considered and removed. Thus, all collars, harnesses or coats should be removed if these are likely to impinge on the part being examined. The feet of animals should always be examined prior to radiography of the extremities, and mud, grit and (in the case of farm animals) stones removed. Similarly it is usually advisable to remove the shoe before radiography of the pedal and navicular bones of the horse. With long-coated sheep, the wool may cast a comparatively dense radiographic shadow, and in some instances in this species clipping is necessary before a satisfactory radiograph can be produced. Light bandages or thin layers of cotton wool around a limb will not affect the radiographic image, but splints and plaster casts should, if possible, be removed before radiography. (Bear in mind that, after the removal of plaster casts, many fragments of plaster may remain attached to the hairs unless thoroughly cleansed.) If the cast or splint may not be removed, the exposure time will have to be increased (see p. 117).

Exposure factors

The large number of different X-ray machines which are now available for veterinary use vary considerably in radiographic output. This fact, together with the wide choice of film and screen combinations make it virtually impossible to suggest suitable exposure factors for each of the examinations described and this information is no longer provided. It will be necessary, therefore, for the veterinary radiographer to complete his own exposure chart in relation to his own apparatus and technique (see Chapter 7). Blank spaces have again been left on each page so that once established, this information can be inserted and is readily available for each examination.

The exposure factors which the authors have found suitable when using particular X-ray machines to undertake the examinations are again included (pp. 355–366).

FORELIMB

1　Scapula

CAUDOCRANIAL (POSTEROANTERIOR)

The animal is placed on its back with both limbs drawn forward and secured with tapes. The chest should be rotated away from the scapula under examination in order to prevent overlap of the radiographic shadow of the rib cage; (This positioning is only practicable when the dog is completely relaxed, and general anaesthesia is normally required.)

Centre through the mid point of the scapula.

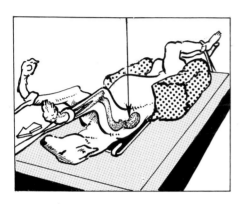

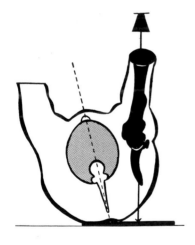

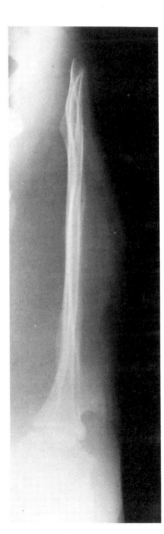

Exposure factors					
Weight	kV	mA	Sec	Grid	Notes
5 kg					
20 kg					
40 kg					

Film type:　　　　　Screen type:　　　　　　　　FFD:

LATERAL

The animal lies on the affected side; the lower forelimb is drawn backwards, while the upper limb is flexed and pulled towards the head.

The central ray is directed perpendicularly to the centre of the scapula. This thin bone is best visualized when superimposed on the lung fields. The dorsal border is often obscured by the vertebrae and if this area is required the thorax must be slightly rotated.

1 Scapula

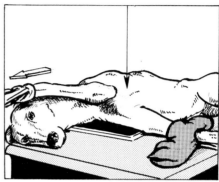

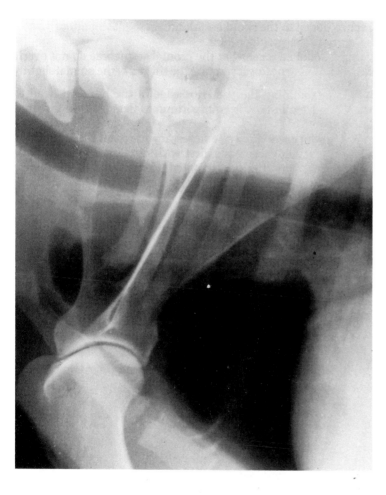

Exposure factors					
Weight 5 kg 20 kg 40 kg	kV	mA	Sec	Grid	Notes

Film type: Screen type: FFD:

3 Humerus

CAUDOCRANIAL (POSTEROANTERIOR)

The dog is placed in dorsal recumbency with both forelegs pulled forwards as for the CdCr scapula view. Centre to the mid-point of the humerus.

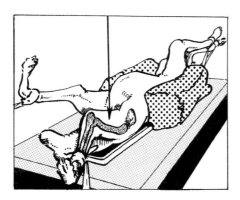

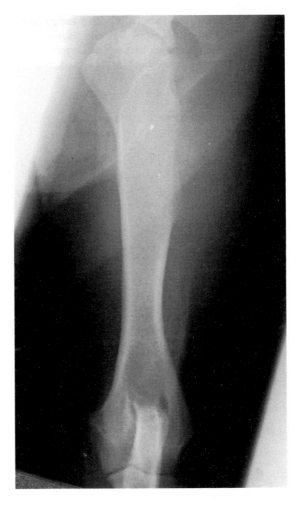

Exposure factors					
Weight	kV	mA	Sec	Grid	Notes
5 kg					
20 kg					
40 kg					

Film type: Screen type: FFD:

LATERAL

The dog is placed on its side with the affected limb down and the humerus resting on the plate. The limb is slightly extended and the upper limb is drawn caudally and secured.
    The beam is directed vertically to the centre of the humerus.

3   Humerus

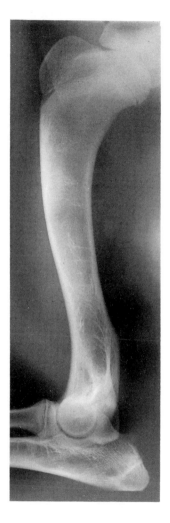

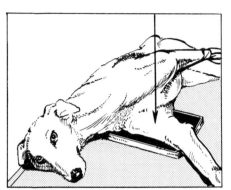

Exposure factors						
Weight	kV	mA	'	Sec	Grid	Notes
5 kg						
20 kg						
40 kg						

Film type: Screen type: FFD:

4 Elbow Joint

CRANIOCAUDAL (ANTEROPOSTERIOR)

The animal is placed in sternal recumbency with both forelimbs extended cranially. Care should be taken to prevent the affected elbow from sliding laterally. A foam pad under the point of the elbow can often help to prevent this. The dog's head should be positioned away from the affected side. Centre through the humero-radial joint.

A caudocranial view can be taken with the animal in dorsal recumbency and both forelegs pulled forwards, as for the CdCr scapula view. Centre through the humero-radial joint. This view will produce some magnification of the image due to the increased object–film distance.

OBLIQUES

Oblique views can be obtained by rotating the affected elbow inwards or outwards. These can be useful to demonstrate peri-articular changes.

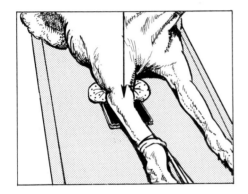

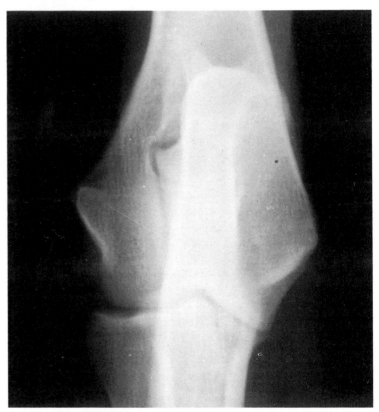

Exposure factors				
Weight	kV	mA	Sec	Notes
5 kg				
20 kg				
40 kg				

Film type:　　　　Screen type:　　　　　　　FFD:

LATERAL

The animal is placed with the affected limb down. For the extended view the limb is drawn cranially and held with a sand bag over the carpus. The head and neck are extended and held in position with another sand bag under the chin. Centre to the medial epicondyle at the lower end of the humerus.

For the flexed view, to demonstrate the anconeal process of the ulna, the projection should be repeated with the elbow fully flexed. It is usually necessary to rotate the chest away from the affected joint with foam wedges under the sternum.

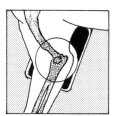
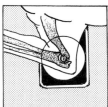

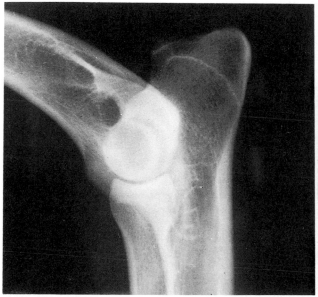
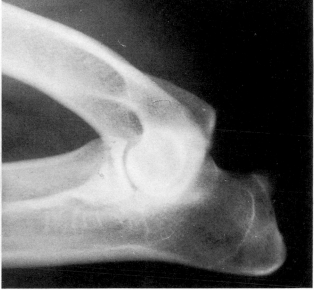

Exposure factors				
Weight	kV	mA	Sec	Notes
5 kg				
20 kg				
40 kg				

Film type: Screen type: FFD:

5 Radius and Ulna

CRANIOCAUDAL (ANTEROPOSTERIOR)

To bring the limb into the correct position it should be pulled forwards with a foam pad under the elbow to prevent rotation at this point. The head is positioned away from the affected limb.
  Centre to the mid-point of the radius and ulna.

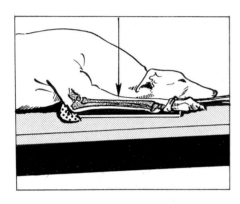

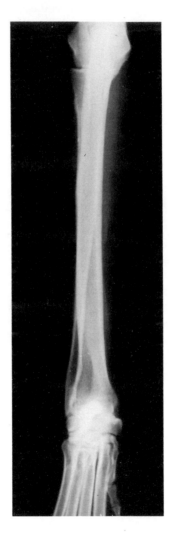

Exposure factors				
Weight	kV	mA	Sec	Notes
5 kg				
20 kg				
40 kg				

Film type: Screen type: FFD:

LATERAL

The animal lies laterally recumbent on the affected side with the upper limb drawn back out of the way. The affected limb can be held in position with a sandbag over the metacarpus.

Direct the central ray to the mid-point of the radius and ulna.

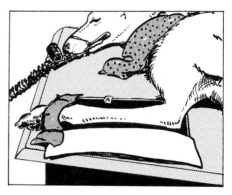

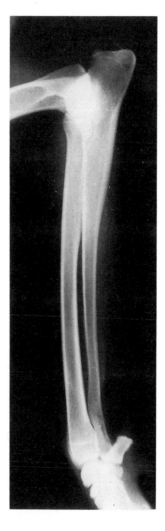

Exposure factors				
Weight	kV	mA	Sec	Notes
5 kg				
20 kg				
40 kg				

Film type: Screen type: FFD:

6 Carpus

INTRODUCTION

Minor injuries are often difficult to detect radiologically, and as well as the standard DPa and lateral views, it may be helpful in doubtful cases, to take both dorsomedial–palmarolateral oblique (anteroposterior–mediolateral oblique) and dorsolateral–palmaromedial oblique (anteroposterior–lateromedial oblique) views.

Comparison views of the sound limb are frequently of value, especially in young and chondrodystrophic breeds.

The use of a small cone and high definition screens will improve the detail.

Views to show individual carpal bones to the best advantage

Carpal	Views in order of importance		
	1	2	3
Proximal row			
radial carpal	DPa	DL-PaMO	Lateral
ulnar carpal	DM-PaLO	DPa	Lateral
accessory carpal	Lateral	DL-PaMO	DPa
Distal row			
first	DL-PaMO	DM-PaLO	DPa
second	DPa	DM-PaLO	—
third	DPa	—	—
fourth	DL-PaMO	DPa	—

DORSOPALMAR (ANTEROPOSTERIOR)

The animal is placed prone with the carpus flat upon the plate. Rotation is prevented by a soft pad under the elbow.

   Where comparative DPa views of the joints are to be made, each carpus must be radiographed separately.

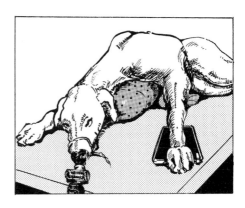

6 Carpus

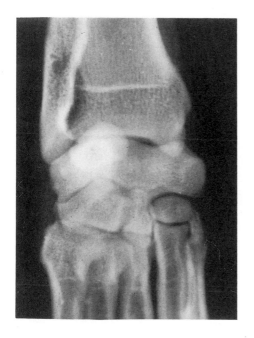

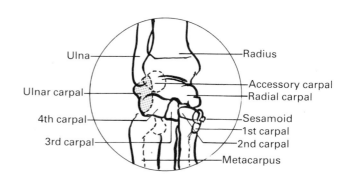

Exposure factors				
Weight	kV	mA	Sec	Notes
5 kg				
20 kg				
40 kg				

Film type: Screen type: FFD:

6 Carpus

DORSOLATERAL–PALMAROMEDIAL OBLIQUE (ANTEROPOSTERIOR–LATEROMEDIAL OBLIQUE)

With the animal in sternal recumbency, the forelimb under investigation is rotated inwards until the carpus lies in a plane at 45° to the film. Foam pads should be used under the elbow and head to facilitate the correct angle. Sedation or general anaesthesia is necessary to permit adequate positioning without holding the limb.

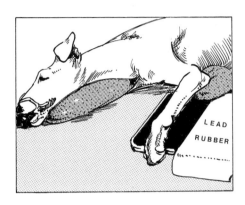

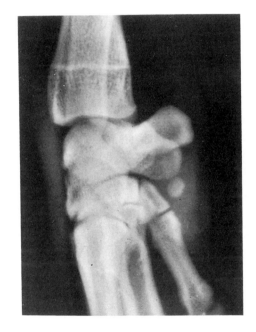

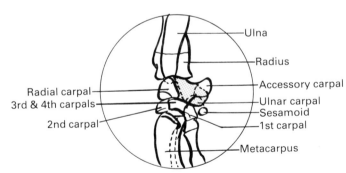

Exposure factors				
Weight	kV	mA	Sec	Notes
5 kg				
20 kg				
40 kg				

Film type: Screen type: FFD:

DORSOMEDIAL–PALMAROLATERAL OBLIQUE
(ANTEROPOSTERIOR–MEDIOLATERAL OBLIQUE)

6 Carpus

The animal is placed in sternal recumbency with a sand bag against the chest on the affected side to allow outward rotation of the foreleg. The limb is pulled cranially by means of a tape to maintain an angle of 45° at the carpus. The head and neck are positioned away from the limb under investigation. Sedation or general anaesthesia is necessary to prevent the need to hold the limb.

Centre to the carpus.

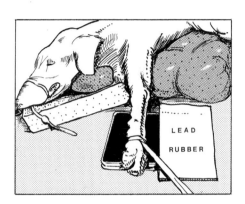

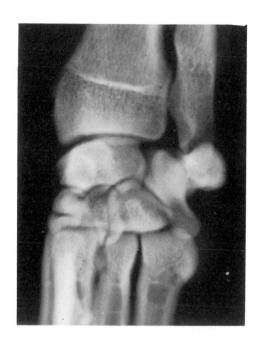

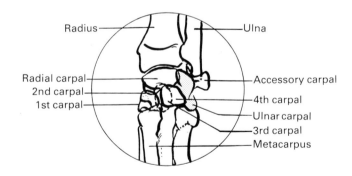

Exposure factors				
Weight 5 kg 20 kg 40 kg	kV mA Sec			Notes

Film type: Screen type: FFD:

6 Carpus

LATERAL

The animal lies laterally recumbent with the affected side down. A foam pad under the elbow helps prevent rotation at the carpus, which should be extended for this view.

Centre to the carpus.

FLEXED LATERAL

In certain conditions, it may be useful to repeat this view with the carpus in flexion rather than extension.

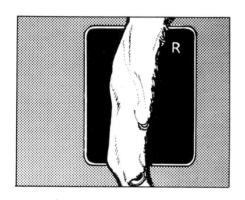

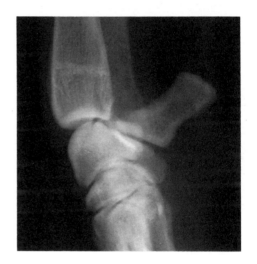

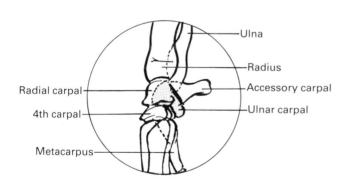

Radial carpal
4th carpal
Metacarpus

Ulna
Radius
Accessory carpal
Ulnar carpal

Exposure factors				
Weight 5 kg 20 kg 40 kg	kV mA Sec			Notes

Film type: Screen type: FFD:

DORSOPALMAR (ANTEROPOSTERIOR)

The animal lies prone with the foot flat upon the plate, as indicated under Carpus. Centre to the middle of the metacarpus.

Normally, to get comparative views of both fore-feet it is necessary to make two exposures.

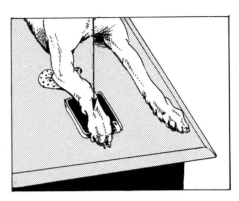

7 Metacarpus

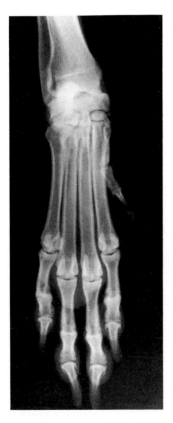

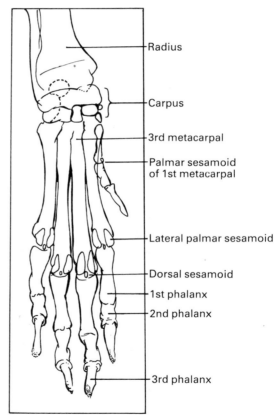

- Radius
- Carpus
- 3rd metacarpal
- Palmar sesamoid of 1st metacarpal
- Lateral palmar sesamoid
- Dorsal sesamoid
- 1st phalanx
- 2nd phalanx
- 3rd phalanx

Exposure factors				
Weight 5 kg 20 kg 40 kg	kV	mA	Sec	Notes

Film type: Screen type: FFD:

7 Metacarpus

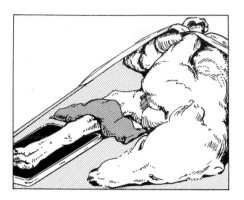

LATERAL

The position illustrated needs little comment. Centre to the middle of the region and always include the carpal joint.

OBLIQUE

Because of superimposition, the value of the lateral view is limited. If it is desired to open out the individual metacarpals, the beam should be angled across the long axis of the foot at roughly 30° to the vertical.

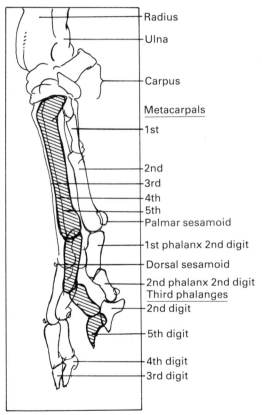

- Radius
- Ulna
- Carpus

Metacarpals
- 1st
- 2nd
- 3rd
- 4th
- 5th
- Palmar sesamoid
- 1st phalanx 2nd digit
- Dorsal sesamoid
- 2nd phalanx 2nd digit

Third phalanges
- 2nd digit
- 5th digit
- 4th digit
- 3rd digit

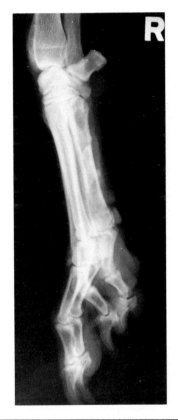

Exposure factors				
Weight 5 kg 20 kg 40 kg	kV	mA	Sec	Notes

Film type: Screen type: FFD:

DORSOPALMAR (ANTEROPOSTERIOR)

The positioning and exposure factors are the same as for DPa metacarpus.

The digits can be flattened by pressing down with a strip of radiolucent adhesive tape.

LATERAL

Some difficulty may be experienced with the digits due to superimposition.

It is often necessary to isolate the affected digit with two bands of bandage, as illustrated.

N.B. If examining the paw for small foreign bodies it is essential to make sure that the screens are clean to avoid artifacts.

8   Digits

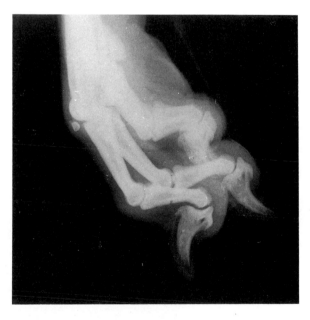

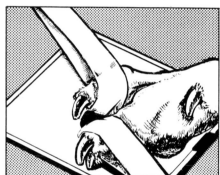

Exposure factors				
Weight 5 kg 20 kg 40 kg	kV mA Sec			Notes

Film type: Screen type: FFD:

HINDLIMB

9 Pelvis

INTRODUCTION

The pelvic area includes the lumbo-sacral junction, sacrum and anterior coccyx, both os coxae and both upper femora. Special views of the vertebrae will be dealt with under *spine*. The os coxa consists of the ilium, ischium and pubis, and all three bones help to form the acetabulum. Because these bones are well demonstrated in all the projections of the more important hip joint, it is not necessary to describe them separately.

The ventrodorsal view of the pelvis with legs in extension provides the best view for evaluation of the hips and pelvis. If pain is experienced on extension of the limbs then the ventrodorsal view can be taken with the hindlimbs in flexion. The lateral view of the pelvis provides some additional information but because of superimposition is not helpful for evaluating the hip joints. The lateral view with an oblique beam will separate the hip joints and is useful in assessing reduction of a dislocated hip.

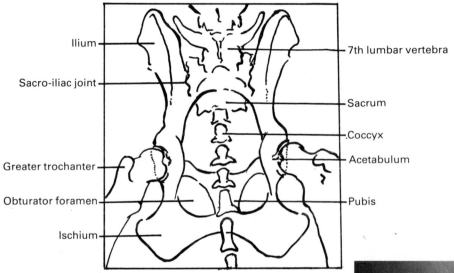

Ilium —
Sacro-iliac joint —
Greater trochanter —
Obturator foramen —
Ischium —
— 7th lumbar vertebra
— Sacrum
— Coccyx
— Acetabulum
— Pubis

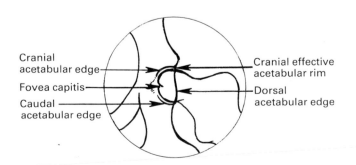

Cranial acetabular edge —
Fovea capitis —
Caudal acetabular edge —
— Cranial effective acetabular rim
— Dorsal acetabular edge

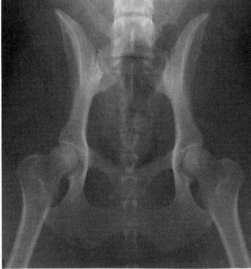

VENTRODORSAL: LEGS IN EXTENSION

This is generally accepted as the standard projection for the pelvic area and for evaluation of the hips for hip dysplasia.

The animal lies upon its back supported by a trough. The pelvis and femora must be included on the film. It is most important that the animal should be bilaterally symmetrical. The hindlegs are extended and secured by tapes so that the femora are parallel to the table top. The stifles are inwardly rotated and held in position by a bandage with the patellae centred between the femoral condyles. This manoeuvre also hyperextends the spine and brings the long axis of the pelvis parallel to the film. Any tilting of the pelvis will give a false illusion of depth to the acetabulae.

For some animals the precise positioning required for the hip dysplasia scheme necessitates the hindlegs being held manually. In these cases the gloved hands should be well outside the primary beam and further protected by a lead rubber shield.

Centre to the cranial border of the pubic symphysis. The X-ray field should include the patellae which should be over the midlines of the femora.

For films intended to be submitted for hip dysplasia certification, the use of sedation or general anaesthesia to immobilize the dog, the employment of a grid to produce optimum definition, and radiographic or photographic methods of permanent indentification of the radiograph with the specified data, will be required.

9   Pelvis

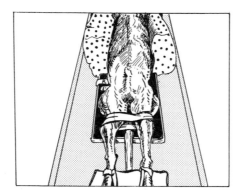

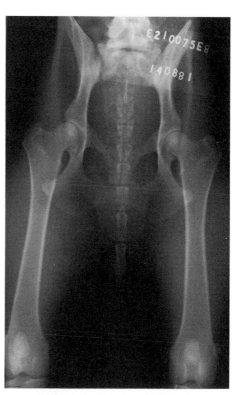

Exposure factors					
Weight	kV	mA	Sec	Grid	Notes
5 kg					
20 kg					
40 kg					

Film type: Screen type: FFD:

9 Pelvis

VENTRODORSAL: LEGS IN FLEXION

This position is more suitable where there is suspected trauma and the patient resents extension, but it is also useful as a second view to confirm pathological changes.

The animal lies on its back in a trough so that it is bilaterally symmetrical. The hind legs are equally flexed and abducted and held in position by a sandbag over the hocks. Care must be taken not to tilt the long axis of the pelvis. A soft pad under the lumbar spine may help to avoid this.

Centre to the cranial border of the pubic symphysis.

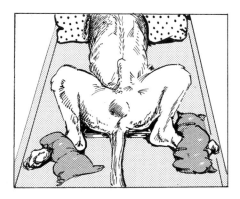

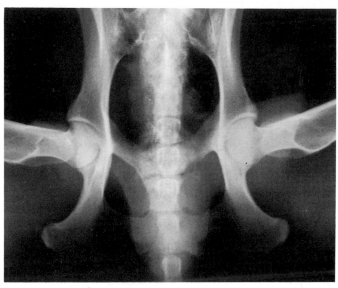

Exposure factors					
Weight	kV	mA	Sec	Grid	Notes
5 kg					
20 kg					
40 kg					

Film type: Screen type: FFD:

LATERAL

The dog is positioned in lateral recumbency. A foam pad of suitable thickness should be placed between the stifles to keep the femora parallel to the cassette. Additional padding may be required under the lumbar spine and under the sternum to prevent rotation.

Centre through the acetabuli.

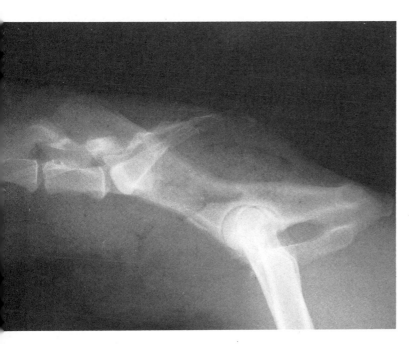

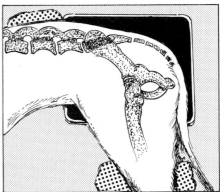

Exposure factors					
Weight	kV	mA	Sec	Grid	Notes
5 kg					
20 kg					
40 kg					

Film type: Screen type: FFD:

9 Pelvis

LATERAL FOR REDUCED DISLOCATED HIP

It is often inadvisable to place any strain on the joint after reduction of a dislocated hip. A lateral hip joint view is useful to confirm reduction.

The animal lies with the reduced joint *uppermost*. The central ray is directed cranially through the uppermost joint at an angle of about 20°. This is to avoid superimposition. If a grid is used care must be taken to angle along its long axis.

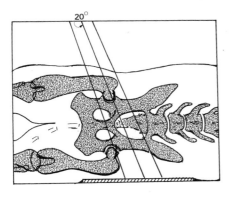

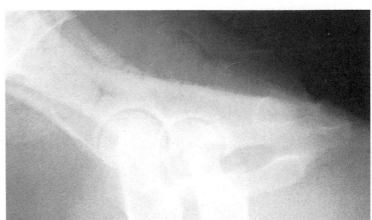

Exposure factors					
Weight	kV	mA	Sec	Grid	Notes
5 kg					
20 kg					
40 kg					

Film type: Screen type: FFD:

VENTRODORSAL

As for VD pelvis, see p. 161.

10 Hip Joint

OBLIQUE LATERAL

The animal is placed in lateral recumbency with the affected side down. In order to ensure that the hip joint is not obscured, the upper limb is pulled back and secured out of the way and the central ray tilted towards the pelvis.

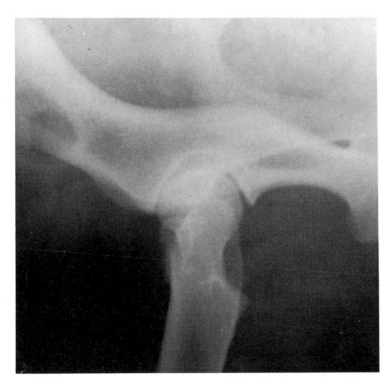

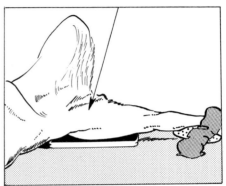

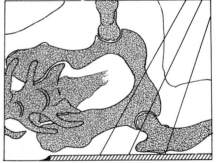

Exposure factors					
Weight	kV	mA	Sec	Grid	Notes
5 kg					
20 kg					
40 kg					

Film type: Screen type: FFD:

11 Femur

CRANIOCAUDAL (ANTEROPOSTERIOR)

The animal lies on its back with both femora extended, as for the VD pelvic view (p. 161). The femur under investigation should be parallel to the film. It is important to rotate the stifle medially so that the patella is centred between the femoral condyles.

Centre to the mid-point of the affected femur.

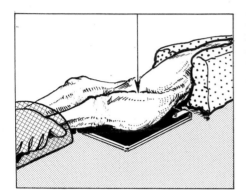

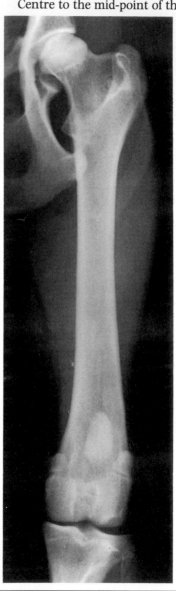

Exposure factors					
Weight	kV	mA	Sec	Grid	Notes
5 kg					
20 kg					
40 kg					

Film type: Screen type: FFD:

LATERAL

The animal lies on the affected side with the opposite limb positioned approximately upright.

Good views of the whole length of the bone are difficult in this projection due to:

(a) The problem of preventing superimposition of the other limb. This can be overcome, particularly in the animal which is tense from nervousness or pain, by sedation or general anaesthesia. Padding under the sternum to rotate the body may also help.

(b) Variation of tissue thickness of the upper and lower limits of the bone. This is most marked in the short-legged breeds and may require two radiographs using different exposure factors to demonstrate the complete femur adequately.

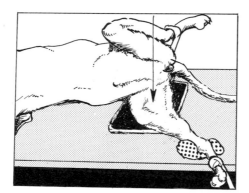

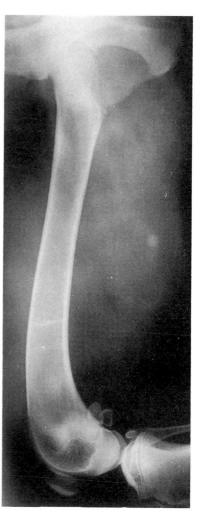

Exposure factors					
Weight 5 kg 20 kg 40 kg	kV	mA	Sec	Grid	Notes

Film type: Screen type: FFD:

11 Femur

ALTERNATIVE LATERAL

The animal lies on the affected side and the affected limb is flexed so that it is covered by the flesh of the abdomen.

The upper femur is gently retracted.

The soft tissues of the abdomen will even out the variation in thickness between lateral hip and lateral stifle. This examination is feasible even where there is severe injury of the femur.

Centre to the middle of the affected femur.

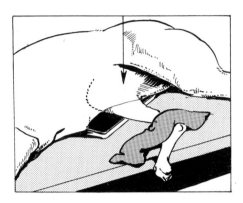

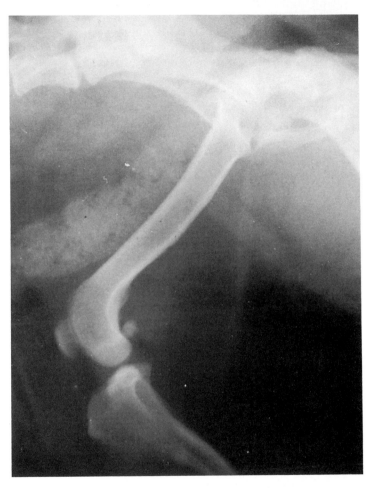

Exposure factors					
Weight	kV	mA	Sec	Grid	Notes
5 kg					
20 kg					
40 kg					

Film type: Screen type: FFD:

CRANIOCAUDAL (ANTEROPOSTERIOR)

This is the most suitable position for radiography of the stifle joint in sedated animals. The animal is positioned in dorsal recumbency with the limb under investigation extended as for the CrCd femoral view (p. 166). Although easier to position than the caudocranial view of the stifle, this view has the disadvantage of some magnification and distortion of the image due to the increased distance between the stifle and the film.

Centre through the stifle joint.

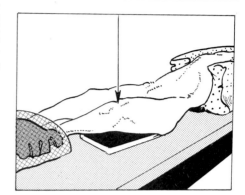

12 Stifle Joint

CAUDOCRANIAL (POSTEROANTERIOR)

The animal is placed in sternal recumbency with both hindlimbs extended posteriorly. The stifle under investigation is rotated medially to centre the patella between the femoral condyles.

Centre through the stifle joint.

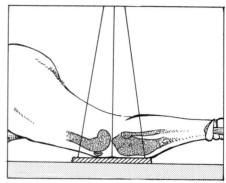

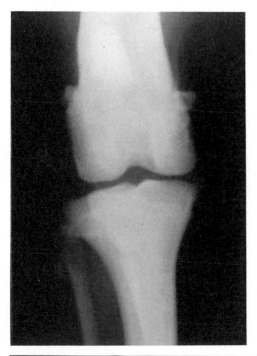

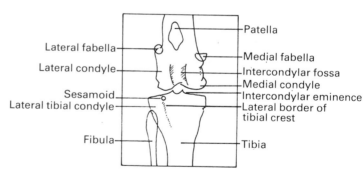

		Patella
Lateral fabella		Medial fabella
Lateral condyle		Intercondylar fossa
		Medial condyle
Sesamoid		Intercondylar eminence
Lateral tibial condyle		Lateral border of tibial crest
Fibula		Tibia

Exposure factors						
Weight	kV	mA	Sec	Grid	Notes	
5 kg						
20 kg						
40 kg						

Film type: Screen type: FFD:

12 Stifle Joint

LATERAL

The true lateral projection of the stifle is essential for accurate diagnosis, but it should not be difficult to achieve in the sedated animal.

The patient lies upon the affected side with the upper hind limb abducted and flexed so that it is out of the way as for the lateral femur. Check that the os penis does not overlie the joint. The stifle under examination should be moderately flexed and not rotated. A soft pad beneath the hock will support the limb and keep the long axis of the tibia parallel to the film. The limb can be maintained in this position with a sandbag over the hock.

The medial tibial condyle is easily palpable and provides a landmark from which to judge the position of the joint space.

Centre vertically to the joint space so that the central ray runs parallel to the surfaces of the tibial condyles.

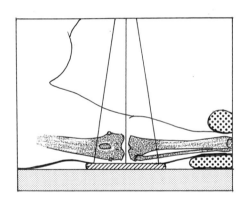

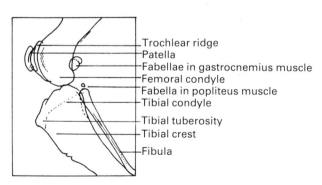

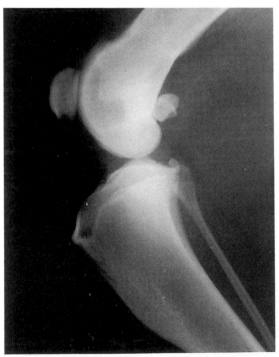

Trochlear ridge
Patella
Fabellae in gastrocnemius muscle
Femoral condyle
Fabella in popliteus muscle
Tibial condyle

Tibial tuberosity
Tibial crest

Fibula

Exposure factors					
Weight 5 kg 20 kg 40 kg	kV	mA	Sec		Notes

Film type: Screen type: FFD:

SKYLINE VIEW OF THE TROCHLEAR GROOVE OF THE FEMUR

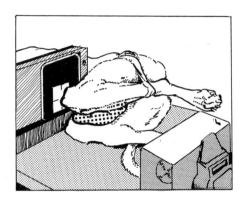

12 Stifle Joint

In certain cases of recurrent dislocating patella, it is necessary to visualize the femoral trochlear groove.

This is most easily achieved with the animal lying on its side with the stifle to be radiographed uppermost, horizontal, fully flexed and supported on a soft pad.

A small film is firmly positioned against the anterior aspect of the thigh at right-angles to the trochlear groove.

The central ray is directed along the groove at right-angles to the film.

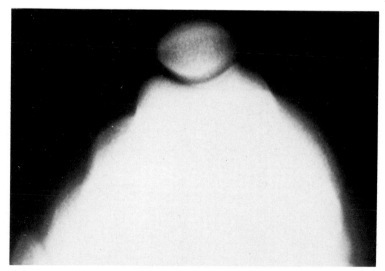

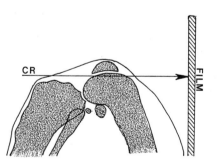

Exposure factors				
Weight 5 kg 20 kg 40 kg	kV	mA	Sec	Notes

Film type: Screen type: FFD:

13 Tibia and Fibula

CRANIOCAUDAL (ANTEROPOSTERIOR)

The animal is placed in dorsal recumbency with the limb under investigation extended posteriorly. It is important to rotate the stifle medially in order to centre the patella between the femoral condyles and to place a foam pad under the metatarsal region to keep the tibia and fibula parallel to the film.

In order to support the trunk in the upright position it may be helpful to flex the opposite limb.

Centre to the mid-point of the tibia and fibula.

A caudocranial view can be taken in the same way as for a caudocranial view of the stifle (p. 169), but centre to the mid-point of the tibia and fibula.

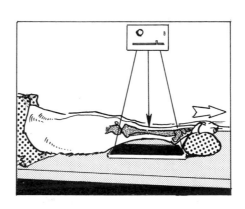

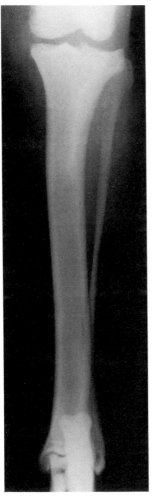

Exposure factors				
Weight 5 kg 20 kg 40 kg	kV	mA	Sec	Notes

Film type: Screen type: FFD:

LATERAL

The animal lies on the affected side with the limb to be radiographed slightly flexed and maintained in the true lateral position by means of a sandbag over the metatarsus. The upper limb is pulled clear by means of tapes.

A film large enough to include both the stifle joint and tarsus joint should be used.

Centre to the middle of the film.

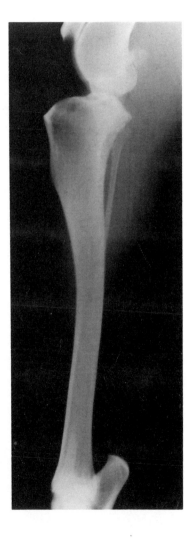

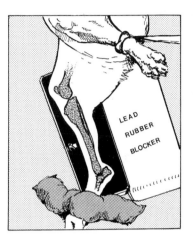

Exposure factors				
Weight 5 kg 20 kg 40 kg	kV mA Sec			Notes

Film type: Screen type: FFD:

14 Tarsus

DORSOPLANTAR (ANTEROPOSTERIOR)

The animal is placed in dorsal recumbency with the limb under investigation extended posteriorly. It is important to make sure the hock is in the true DPl plane by rotating the stifle medially in order to centre the patella between the femoral condyles. The limb should be secured in full extension with a tape. It may be helpful to put a foam pad under the stifle to maintain this position.

Centre through the tarsus.

A plantarodorsal view can be taken using the same position as for the caudocranial stifle (p. 169) but centre through the tarsus.

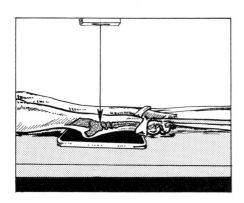

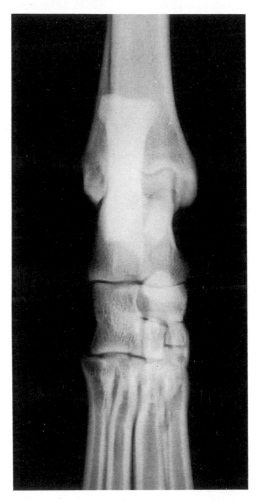

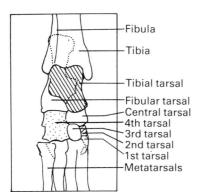

Fibula
Tibia
Tibial tarsal
Fibular tarsal
Central tarsal
4th tarsal
3rd tarsal
2nd tarsal
1st tarsal
Metatarsals

Exposure factors				
Weight	kV	mA	Sec	Notes
5 kg				
20 kg				
40 kg				

Film type: Screen type: FFD:

LATERAL

The animal lies on the affected side with the joint to be radiographed in the centre of the plate and maintained in the true lateral position by a sand bag over the paw.

The upper limb is flexed out of the way of the beam and secured with tapes.

Centre to the tarsus.

OBLIQUE

In order to highlight fine radiographic changes, supplementary oblique views can be obtained by angling the tarsus to the central ray (cf. Carpus, p. 152).

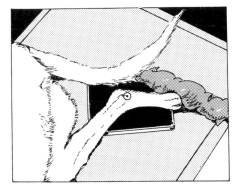

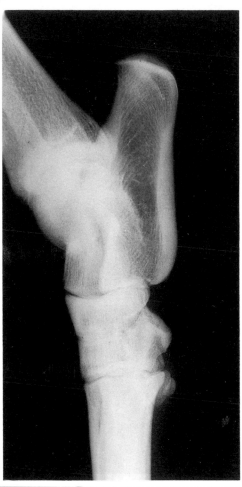

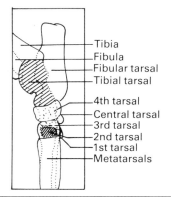

- Tibia
- Fibula
- Fibular tarsal
- Tibial tarsal
- 4th tarsal
- Central tarsal
- 3rd tarsal
- 2nd tarsal
- 1st tarsal
- Metatarsals

Exposure factors				
Weight	kV	mA	Sec	Notes
5 kg				
20 kg				
40 kg				

Film type: Screen type: FFD:

14 Tarsus

16 General

DORSOVENTRAL

This position is more suitable for the sedated animal than the ventrodorsal view.

The animal should rest in a comfortable crouching position. The head is placed on a cassette which, in turn, rests upon a suitable wooden block. Gentle pressure with a sandbag over the neck should bring the head into the dorsoventral position.

The sagittal plane should be vertical, in line with the central ray and at right-angles to the film. The interpupillary line should, therefore, be parallel to the film.

Centre to the mid-point between the eyes.

In certain cases it is helpful if the symphysis rests upon a foam pad.

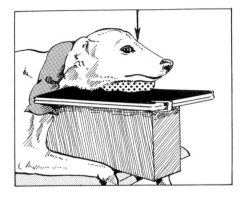

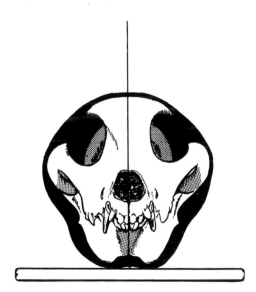

Exposure factors					
Weight 5 kg 20 kg 40 kg	kV	mA	Sec	Grid	Notes

Film type: Screen type: FFD:

VENTRODORSAL

This position is only suitable for anaesthetized or sedated, dolichocephalic breeds. The animal lies upon its back in a trough, with the head and neck extended.

The sagittal plane must be vertical, in line with the central ray and at right-angles to the film.

A soft pad under the neck facilitates positioning of the head. The position can be maintained by means of a tape passed behind the maxillary canine teeth. A foam pad may be placed under the nose.

Centre to the mid-point between the eyes.

16 General

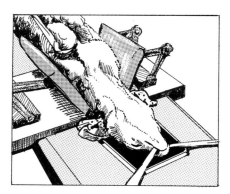

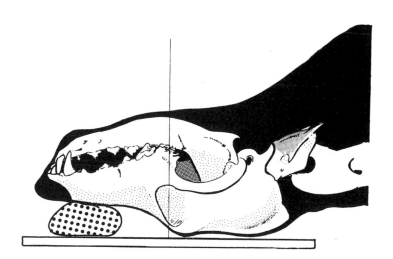

Exposure factors					
Weight	kV	mA	Sec	Grid	Notes
5 kg					
20 kg					
40 kg					

Film type: Screen type: FFD:

16 General

LATERAL

It is possible to radiograph the skull of a conscious animal, but exact superimposition is difficult to achieve without sedation or general anaesthesia. Precise alignment should always be aimed for, because deviation makes interpretation more difficult.

The animal can be placed upon its back and supported in a trough. Allow the trunk to rotate slightly to the affected side and the neck to flex until the head assumes the true lateral position. Maintain the position with soft pads under the neck and muzzle.

Alternatively, the animal can be placed in lateral recumbency and with careful placement of foam wedges under the neck and nose the skull can be brought into the true lateral position.

The sagittal plane should be parallel to the film with the interpupillary line vertical and in line with the central ray.

As the skull is divided into the well aerated nasal chambers and the much denser cranium, exposure will depend upon the region under examination. (Nasal Chambers, see p. 186.)

Centring points:

> *Nasal chambers:* to the middle of the nasal chambers.
> *Cranium:* midway along the orbitomeatal line.

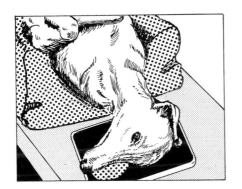

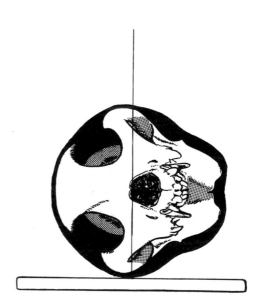

Exposure factors					
Weight	kV	mA	Sec	Grid	Notes
5 kg					
20 kg					
40 kg					

Film type: Screen type: FFD:

16 General

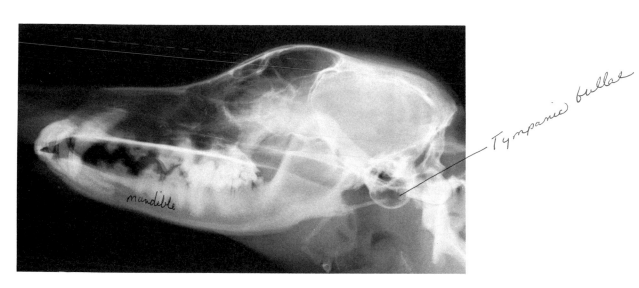

Tympanic bullae

mandible

ETHMOIDAL FOSSAE
FRONTAL SINUSES　　　ZYGOMATIC ARCHES
ORBITS　　　HYPOPHYSEAL FOSSA
MAXILLARY SINUSES　　　CRANIAL CAVITY
NASAL CHAMBERS　　　NUCHAL CREST
OCCIPITAL CONDYLES

MANDIBLE
PALATINE PROCESS　　　FORAMEN MAGNUM
CAUDAL NARES　　　TYMPANIC BULLAE
SOFT PALATE　　　EXT. AUDITORY MEATUSES
HYOID APPARATUS　　　TEMPOROMANDIBULAR JOINTS

23 Lower Jaw

PREMOLAR AND MOLAR TEETH: DORSOVENTRAL 45° OBLIQUE

When an assessment of the mandibular arcade is made on a sedated animal, the oblique view described for the maxillary molars (p. 195) will usually suffice. However it should be recognized that the tooth roots most clearly seen in this view are those furthest from the film. If a ventrodorsal 45° oblique view is used the tooth roots nearest the film will be shown most accurately.

PREMOLAR AND MOLAR TEETH—LATERAL INTRAORAL

The most accurate visualization of the mandibular molar teeth is obtained by inserting a small non-screen 'dental' film against the medial border of the mandible. The animal is positioned, lying on its side with the teeth to be examined uppermost. The film is maintained in position, held with a pair of forceps. The mandible and film are positioned so that they are at 90° to the vertical central ray. Centre on the affected tooth.

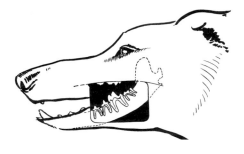

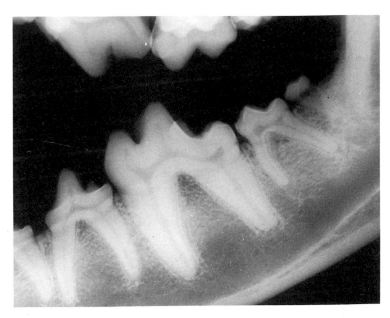

Exposure factors				
Weight 5 kg 20 kg 40 kg	kV	mA	Sec	Notes

Film type: Screen type: FFD:

INTRODUCTION

Radiographically, the spine can be divided into the following areas:

Cervical	C1–C6
Cervico-thoracic	C6–T3
Thoracic	T3–T11
Thoraco-lumbar	T11–L3
Lumbar	L1–L7
Sacrum and cranial coccyx	L7–Cy3–4

The differences in tissue thickness are not significant in cats and small dogs under 9 kg (20 lb) in weight, but in larger animals the difference in radiopacity of these regions necessitates different exposure factors.

General positioning

Apart from gross traumatic injury, the diagnosis of spinal lesions such as disc protrusions, bone changes and calcification within the neural canal depends upon good positioning and the demonstration of fine detail. Accurate positioning can only be obtained in painful conditions with general anaesthesia. A grid or high definition screens and close collimation of the beam are desirable.

The principles of positioning the spine discussed on the next two pages are applicable to all areas.

SPINE

24 General

24 General

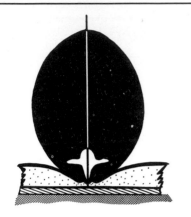

VENTRODORSAL

It is difficult to position a thin animal in the ventrodorsal position, but a foam rubber pad will make it more comfortable.

The sagittal plane must be vertical and in line with the central ray.

Apart from the cervical spine, which must be extended, the animal should be positioned with the vertebral column in the natural slightly flexed position. The hind legs should not be over-extended; the femora should be vertical and slightly abducted.

LATERAL

The long axis of the spine does not normally lie parallel to the table top when an animal is laterally recumbent, so soft pads must usually be placed under the head, neck, lumbar spine and pelvis. The sagittal plane through the vertebrae should also be parallel to the film. This is achieved by keeping the upper legs parallel to the top of the table and padding underneath the sternum.

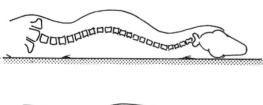

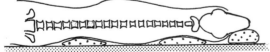

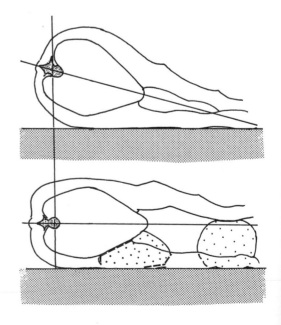

INTERVERTEBRAL DISC INVESTIGATION

Where interverbral disc lesions are suspected a more critical technique must be used. A general lateral view of the area should first be taken and examined. In medium- and larger-sized animals it is usual to find that only a few intervertebral spaces around the centring point appear open, while those at the edge of the film are distorted by the spreading beam and appear progressively narrowed. The vertebrae are not close to the film and, even in a small animal, some magnification and distortion will occur. The general lateral view should indicate any suspicious area and a localized 'coned down' view should be taken next, the central ray being directed to the queried disc space. The exact localization can be made from measurements made on the general lateral view, using a fixed point, such as the iliac crest.

24 General

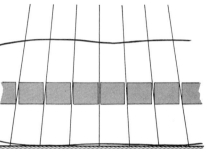

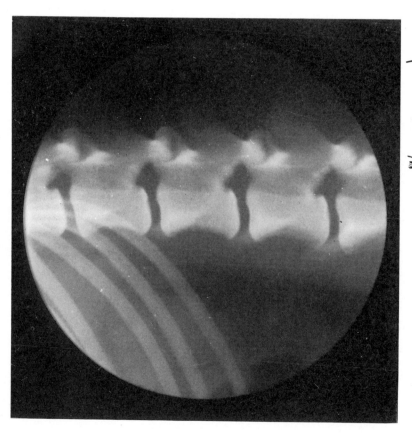

25 Cervical Spine (C1–C6)

VENTRODORSAL

The animal lies upon its back with the head and neck extended so that the cervical spine lies roughly parallel to the film. A tape around the muzzle will secure the head in this position.

The angle of the vertebral bodies makes it necessary to angle the central ray about 15° to the head, in the midline, midway between the shoulders and the base of skull. If a grid is used be sure to angle the beam along the lines of the grid.

General anaesthesia is necessary to achieve adequate relaxation. Any endotracheal tube will be superimposed on the vertebral bodies and should be removed prior to making the exposure.

The open mouth view to show the tympanic bullae will also demonstrate very clearly the odontoid process and the atlanto-axial articulation (p. 191).

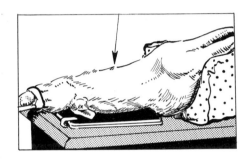

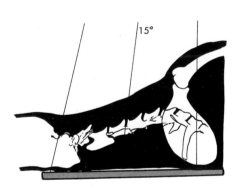

Exposure factors					
Weight	kV	mA	Sec	Grid	Notes
5 kg					
20 kg					
40 kg					

Film type: Screen type: FFD:

LATERAL

The animal lies upon its side. The forelegs are pulled well back, the neck extended and gentle traction exerted. Care must be taken to keep lead protected hands away from the primary beam, the extent of which can only be satisfactorily judged with a light beam diaphragm.

The spine must be parallel to the film, and foam packing under the neck and muzzle will be necessary.

If the animal is in pain, anaesthesia will be necessary to achieve relaxation. Close collimation will enhance detail.

Centre vertically to the spine over the suspected area.

Hyperflexed and hyperextended views can be of value, especially when combined with myelography to detect cervical stenosis and spondylolisthesis.

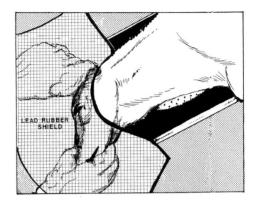

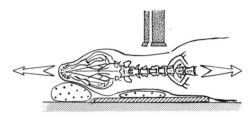

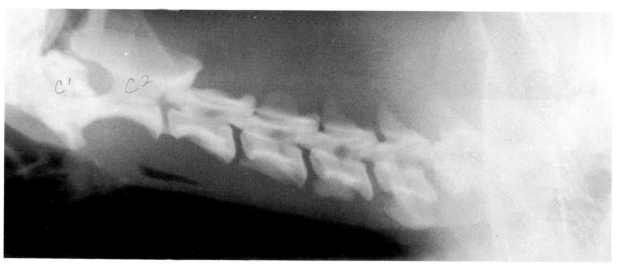

Exposure factors					
Weight	kV	mA	Sec	Grid	Notes
5 kg					
20 kg					
40 kg					

Film type: Screen type: FFD:

29 Sacrum

VENTRODORSAL

The animal lies in a trough on its back with the legs extended. The pelvis must be symmetrically placed upon the film.

The central ray is directed at 30° to the head through the sacrum in the midline.

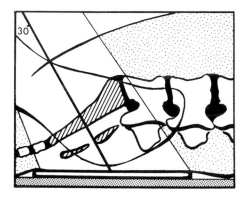

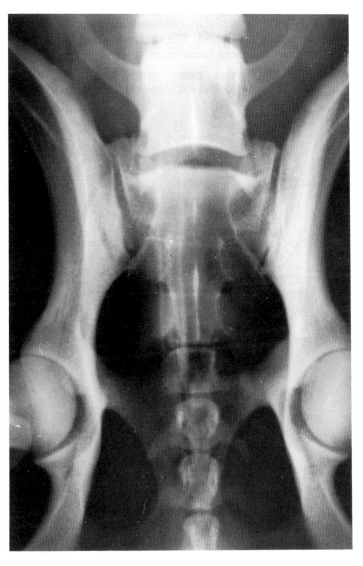

Exposure factors					
Weight 5 kg 20 kg 40 kg	kV mA	Sec	Grid	Notes	

Film type: Screen type: FFD:

LATERAL

29 Sacrum

The animal lies upon its side with the spine parallel to the table-top. The hind-legs are moderately extended and padded so that the pelvis is not tilted.

Centre to the body of the sacrum.

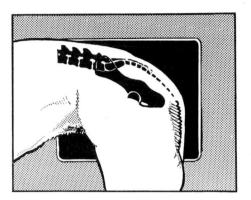

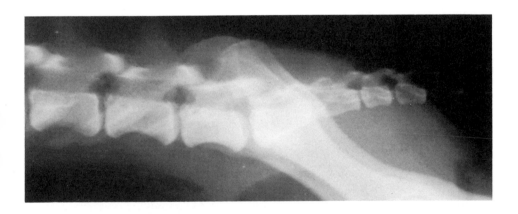

Exposure factors						
Weight	kV	mA	Sec	Grid	Notes	
5 kg						
20 kg						
40 kg						

Film type: Screen type: FFD:

30 Coccyx

DORSOVENTRAL

The animal is placed in sternal or dorsal recumbency with its tail extended backwards and resting on high definition screens or non-screen film, supported on a wooden block. The central ray is directed vertically to the centre of the tail.

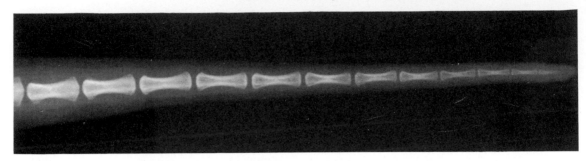

LATERAL

The animal lies upon its side with the tail extended backwards across high definition screens or non-screen film resting on a wooden block. Centre to the middle of the tail.

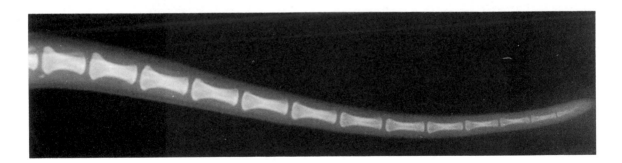

Exposure factors				
Weight	kV	mA	Sec	Notes
5 kg				
20 kg				
40 kg				

Film type: Screen type: FFD:

The general term 'soft tissues' is used here to include the muscular system and adjacent tissues, the pharynx and associated structures and the thoracic and abdominal cavities and their respective contents.

The main problem in soft tissue radiography is the fact that there are only slight differences in the radiodensity of the various tissues, and it is therefore very difficult to produce a good 'contrasty' radiograph. Exposure factors must be selected with care, and all precautions likely to aid definition (the avoidance of movement, collimation, the use of grids for dense areas, etc.) should be employed. The use of contrast agents to facilitate the visualization of a particular organ is described in Chapter 13.

The indications for radiography of the muscular system are very limited, and the two main reasons for undertaking this are:

(a) to show the presence of foreign bodies;
(b) to demonstrate calcification of muscle, tendon or glandular tissue.

Owing to the wide variation in the parts of the muscular system which may need to be radiographed no precise instructions can be given, but the following points should be of assistance:

1   Position the animal according to the instructions given for the part of the skeletal system nearest to the tissue to be examined.
2   Take radiographs in two planes.
3   Exposure factors may be taken from those found suitable for the skeletal system—using the same kV but reducing the mA-s by at least one half, to give a 'softer' radiograph.

Chapter 11

Canine Radiography: Soft Tissues

1 The Muscular System

THE DEMONSTRATION AND LOCALIZATION OF FOREIGN
BODIES

The radiographic demonstration of foreign bodies within areas of
soft tissue will depend on the radiopacity of the object and whether
it is significantly different from the opacity of surrounding tissues.
Metal or stone will be readily apparent, but glass, wood and plastic
material may not be distinguishable from soft tissues. In some
circumstances the presence of air or gas pockets associated with
the foreign bodies may be recognized. Unless the objects are particularly radiopaque, good radiographic technique is essential and,
as mentioned already, exposure factors should be selected so as to
produce softer, less contrasty radiographs. It is also important to
check that suspicious shadows seen on the radiograph are not
caused by marks on the intensifying screens or dirt in the coat.

Localization of a foreign body will depend on the degree of
precision required. For most purposes the position of the object
can be deduced from the examination of two radiographs of the
area taken at right angles to each other. The use of radiopaque
markers attached to the skin or inserted into any associated sinus
before radiography may also help to pinpoint the position of the
foreign body.

Techniques by which the depth of an object beneath the skin
can be calculated have been devised and one such procedure is
described opposite. In general, these methods are of theoretical
rather than practical value.

PROCEDURE FOR ESTIMATING THE DEPTH OF A FOREIGN
BODY BENEATH THE SKIN

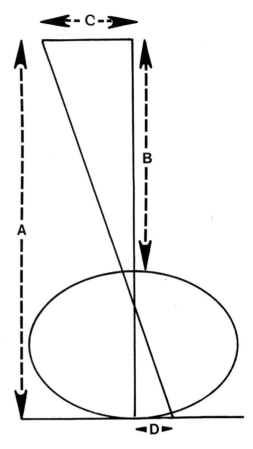

1 Place the patient on the X-ray table and take a survey radiograph to locate the object.
2 Mark the skin immediately above the estimated position of the foreign body.
3 Position the X-ray set directly above the object.
4 Measure accurately the distance from the focal spot to the film (A), and the mark on the skin (B).
5 Make an X-ray exposure using half the normal mA-s.
6 Without shifting the patient or the film cassette, move the X-ray tube a measured distance (10–15 cm) to one side.
7 Repeat the previous exposure.
8 Process the film. This should now show a double image of the foreign body.
9 Measure the displacement of the foreign body. If this displacement is too small for significant measurement either:
    (a) Increase the displacement of the tube.
    or
    (b) Assume that the object is too close to the film and repeat the whole procedure after turning the patient on to its other side.
10 The distance of the foreign body beneath the skin can now be calculated from the formula $\dfrac{AC}{C+D} - B$ when:

  A = the focal–film distance
  B = the focal–skin distance
  C = the movement of the tube
  D = the movement of the image of the foreign body

2   Pharynx

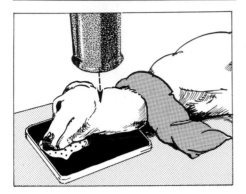

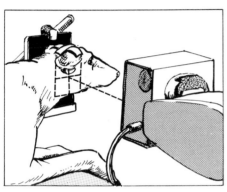

LATERAL

The air passages of the upper respiratory tract act as a contrast agent and permit the soft structures of the pharyngeal area to be visualized. The lateral view is the most informative. The cervical spine obscures detail in the other plane and restricts its usefulness to the locating of foreign bodies.

The animal lies on its side with the forelegs retracted. The head and neck are extended and placed in the true lateral position. The larynx should be clear of the mandible. Centre to the pharynx.

STANDING LATERAL

If it is desired to show the natural relationship between the epiglottis and the soft palate a lateral radiograph should be taken using the horizontal beam with the dog in the standing position. Special care should be taken to observe radiological protection when using the horizontal beam.

Development by inspection is advocated (usually for a reduced time) so that detail of the soft tissue is achieved without producing too much contrast.

Exposure factors					
Weight 5 kg 20 kg 40 kg	kV mA	Sec	Grid	Notes	

Film type: Screen type: FFD:

2 Pharynx

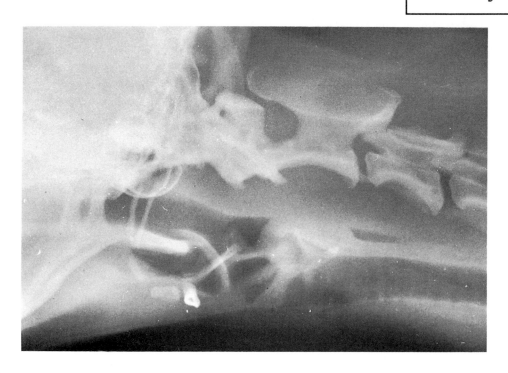

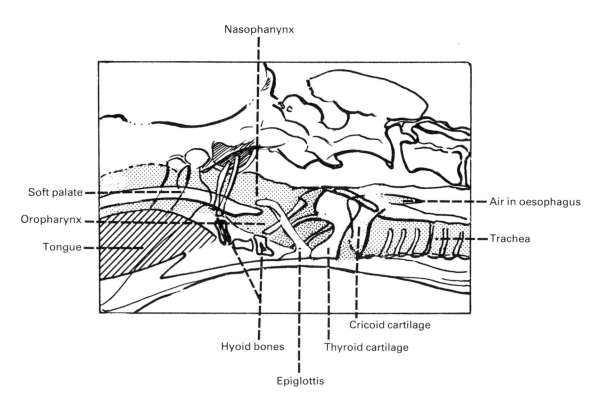

Nasophanynx

Soft palate

Oropharynx

Tongue

Air in oesophagus

Trachea

Cricoid cartilage

Hyoid bones

Thyroid cartilage

Epiglottis

3 Thorax

INTRODUCTION

The production of good radiographs of the thoracic cavity and its contents is one of the most difficult tasks confronting the veterinary radiographer. If this is to be achieved successfully, there are three main requirements to be borne in mind, as described below:

1 The elimination of *movement* (both voluntary and involuntary).
2 The use of as long a *focal–film distance* as is practicable.
3 Precise *positioning* of the patient.

Movement

Voluntary movement of the patient must be checked by careful and comfortable positioning of the patient, adequate control of the animal and, where necessary, the use of sedation or general anaesthesia.

Elimination of involuntary movement (i.e. respiration) may be undertaken in one of two ways.

(a) Exposure times of 0.02–0.04 second are required to eliminate the effect of respiratory movement. Except for the smallest patients, this will necessitate the use of more powerful apparatus or faster film–screen combinations. Rare earth screens have been particularly helpful in this respect.

(b) General anaesthesia can be used to reduce the effect of respiratory movement. With this method it is usual to compress the rebreathing bag in order to hold the lungs at full inspiration while making the exposure. The lungs should not be overinflated but adequate distention with air will help in producing maximum detail and contrast in the finished radiograph.

However, the apparatus necessary for (*a*) may not be available in general practice, and in some instances (*b*) may be considered to involve an unnecessary risk to the patient. Although respiration cannot be controlled, useful radiographs of the chest can often be obtained with portable X-ray apparatus, at least in the smaller patient, provided that attention is paid to the other details of technique to be described, but there will inevitably be some respiratory blur.

When radiographing the chest of an animal in which respirations are unchecked, care should be taken to see that the exposure is made at the same stage of respiration each time— preferably at full inspiration.

A rough-and-ready method of checking respiratory movement that is sometimes of help is to have an assistant close the dog's mouth and briefly pinch its nostrils at the time of making the exposure. For animals under general anaesthesia the same level of inspiration should be aimed for in order to produce comparable films.

Focal–film distance

Since there is considerable depth to an animal's thorax, it is not possible to place all parts close to the film. Therefore if radiography of this area is undertaken at the usual focal–film distance of 75 cm or 100 cm (30 or 39 inches) there will be considerable enlargement of the parts of the chest situated furthest away from the film. Unfortunately any increase in the focal–film distance has to be compensated for by increasing the mA-s output of the X-ray apparatus, which is not practicable with the smaller sets. Thus, while a focal–film distance of 120 cm or more (approximately 4 ft) is advisable for chest radiography in the dog (particularly the dorsoventral view), and is possible with the larger type of machine, with the portable sets one has to be content with a focal–film distance of about 75 cm (30 inches) and some distortion of the image is unavoidable.

Positioning

It is recommended that radiography of the canine chest be undertaken in the dorsoventral and lateral planes. Ventrodorsal positioning is less satisfactory because it results in displacement of the heart which can make interpretation difficult. However it may be easier to position the conscious animal for this projection. Extreme caution should be exercised when radiographing animals with respiratory distress since fatalities can occur if such patients are turned on their back. The lateral view is normally taken with the animal lying on its side, so that the forelimbs may be drawn well forward and the shadow of humeri, scapulae and associated muscle removed as far as possible. If the presence of fluid is suspected within the chest, it may be helpful to radiograph the animal in the standing lateral position, and this area of increased density will then be superimposed on the cranial chest.

Of the two views of the chest the dorsoventral one is the most informative, since it permits comparison of the two sides of chest and prevents their superimposition. Unfortunately, owing to the comparative depth of the canine chest, it is far more difficult to position the thorax satisfactorily in this plane, and considerable care must be taken if this is to be done accurately.

Detail and contrast

It has already been emphasized that exposure times of 0.02–0.04 second are needed to eliminate respiratory movement blur. Reducing the mA-s factor can be achieved by using high kV values which has the advantage of ensuring satisfactory penetration of all areas of the thorax as well as producing a well-balanced radiograph with a broad range of contrast. High contrast radiographs where white and black tones predominate should be avoided. A reduction in exposure can also be obtained without any loss of image quality by using rare earth screens.

3   Thorax

DORSOVENTRAL

The animal lies upon its sternum. The fore-legs are equally abducted, pulled forward and restrained so that the sagittal plane is vertical and in line with the central ray. The hind-legs are flexed in the normal crouching position and, if necessary, supported by sandbags to prevent the hind-quarters from rotating. The head and neck must also be kept low to prevent the musculature of the root of the neck from obscuring the lung apices.

Centre in the midline between the most prominent dorsal parts of the scapulae. Exposure should be made on full inspiration.

A grid is useful to improve definition in larger dogs but can lead to unacceptably long exposure times. It is unnecessary to use a grid if the depth of tissue is less than 20 cm.

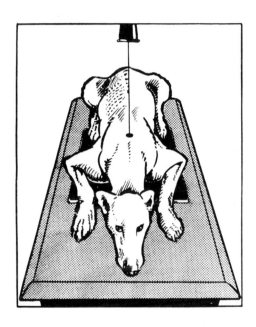

Exposure factors					
Weight	kV	mA	Sec	Grid	Notes
5 kg					
20 kg					
40 kg					

Film type: Screen type: FFD:

DORSOVENTRAL

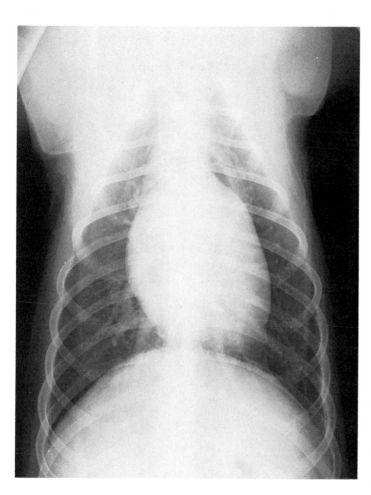

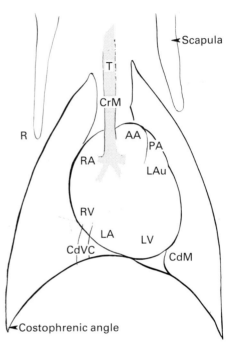

AA	Aortic arch
RA	Right atrium
RV	Right ventricle
PA	Pulmonary artery
LA	Left atrium
LAu	Left auricle
LV	Left ventricle
CrM	Cranial mediastinum
CdM	Ventral caudal mediastinum
CdVC	Caudal vena cava
T	Trachea

3   Thorax

VENTRODORSAL

It is easier to control the uncooperative animal in the ventro-dorsal position, and the positioning of the thorax is aided if the animal lies in a radiolucent trough (see p. 125).

The view is not suitable for the assessment of cardiac pathology because the contour cannot be properly assessed.

Positioning in this plane can be dangerous for the patient in the presence of marked pneumothorax or intrathoracic fluid.

The thorax must be bilaterally symmetrical with the forelegs pulled cranially. The central ray should be directed to the middle of the sternum.

Expose, if possible, at the peak of inspiration.

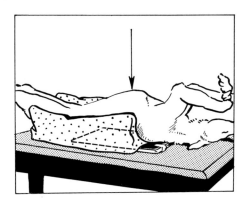

Exposure factors					
Weight	kV	mA	Sec	Grid	Notes
5 kg					
20 kg					
40 kg					

Film type: Screen type: FFD:

VENTRODORSAL

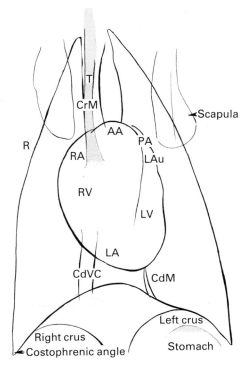

3 Thorax

AA	Aortic arch
RA	Right atrium
RV	Right ventricle
LA	Left atrium
LAu	Left auricle
LV	Left ventricle
PA	Pulmonary artery
CrM	Cranial mediastinum
CdM	Ventral caudal mediastinum
CdVC	Caudal vena cava
T	Trachea

3   Thorax— Demonstration of Fluid Levels

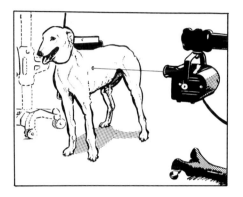

STANDING LATERAL

This position is only used as a means of confirming fluid in the thorax. It is less satisfactory than the recumbent lateral because it is difficult to position the animal accurately and the forelegs obscure the cranial lung fields.

The cassette should be held by a suitable stand and placed as close to the animal as possible.

Centre to the midpoint of the fourth intercostal space.

Exposure factors will be similar to those for the recumbent lateral projection (p. 225), but should be increased if much fluid is present.

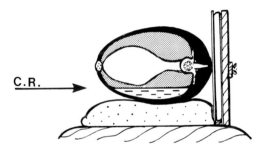

C.R.

RECUMBENT VENTRODORSAL WITH HORIZONTAL BEAM

The animal lies on its side with the forelegs pulled cranially as for a conventional chest film, but on a radiolucent foam pad. The film is aligned vertically and the rays are directed horizontally at the level where a fluid line is expected.

This view is valuable for detecting small amounts of pleural fluid or gas.

Exposure factors					
Weight	kV	mA	Sec	Grid	Notes
5 kg					
20 kg					
40 kg					

Film type: Screen type: FFD:

INTRODUCTION

The main problem in the radiography of the abdominal cavity is the identification and demonstration of a particular organ and its differentiation from other abdominal structures. This is difficult because, not only are the contents of the abdomen variable in position and often superimposed, but they lack the contrast effect of the air which, in the lungs, helps to produce greater definition in the radiograph. In the older, obese animal this lack of air is partly compensated for by the presence of fat which acts as a natural 'contrast agent' and helps to outline the liver and kidneys. Thus one may obtain a radiograph showing better definition of a large but fat animal than of a smaller thin one.

If available a grid should be employed for abdomens greater than 10–15 cm in thickness. The use of a grid will obviously increase exposure time.

Preparation

Except in emergency situations, it is important to ensure that the patient has been starved and has had a recent opportunity to evacuate its bowels and bladder. In some cases a cleansing enema will be required.

Control of movement

Voluntary and involuntary movement must again be controlled; and it is not always realized to what extent respiratory movement can cause blurring of abdominal radiographs. Sedation or general anaesthesia and the use of very short exposure times and faster film–screen combinations help considerably in reducing abdominal movement during radiography. A compression band can help by reducing the depth of tissue but distorts the natural relationship of the abdominal organs.

Positioning

Owing to the comparative mobility of the abdominal organs and of the surrounding abdominal muscle there will always be some displacement of the abdominal contents when the dog is laid on the film cassette, and positioning need not be quite so precise as for the chest. (A lateral radiograph taken with the dog in the standing position might give a slightly more accurate picture of the relative positions of the abdominal organs, but there will be considerable distortion and loss of detail, because the dog cannot be restrained satisfactorily or so closely applied to the film.)

Radiography in the ventrodorsal plane is advised, because this position helps to spread and extend the abdomen; whereas dorso-ventral positioning causes the animal to crouch and to compress the abdomen. Positioning in the former way also makes for easier restraint.

Collimation

If one is concerned with demonstrating a particular organ or area of the abdomen, then in addition to the standard projections, close collimation and centring to the area of interest will help improve definition. This technique is particularly useful when employed in conjunction with contrast studies.

SPINE

The thoracic and lumbar spine is
demonstrated on the next two pages.

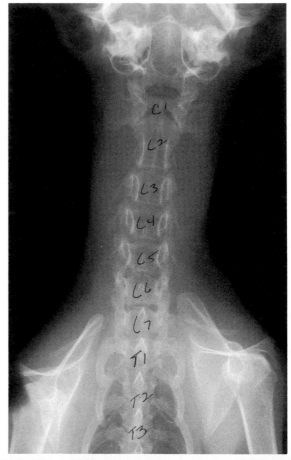

Cervical spine—ventrodorsal

Cervical spine—lateral
(Note clavicle in shoulder area)

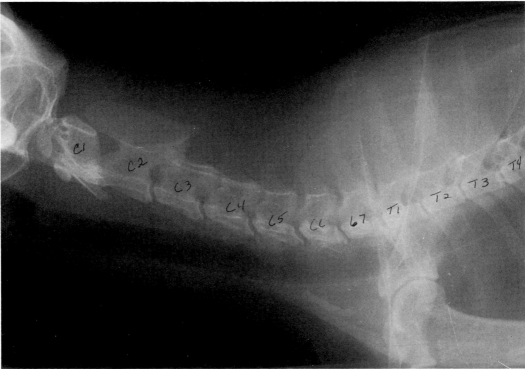

Thorax

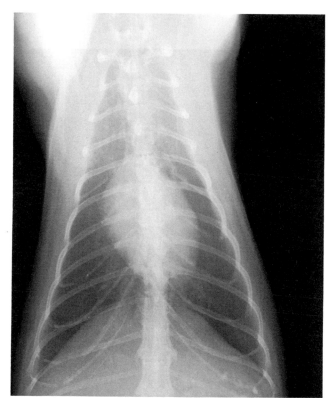

Thorax—dorsoventral

Thorax—lateral

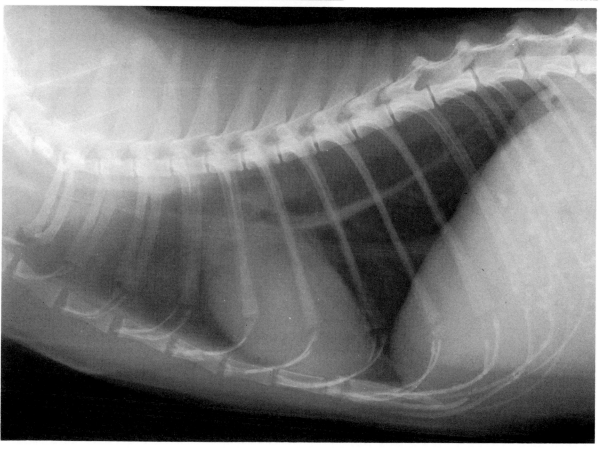

3   to check that the patient has been adequately prepared for the contrast examination
4   to make sure that the contrast technique chosen is the most appropriate to help with the diagnosis
5   to help estimate the amount of contrast media that will be required for the technique.

The principal contrast media techniques employed in veterinary radiography are summarized in subsequent pages. While certain contrast agents which have proved to be of value for particular procedures are mentioned, it is likely that there are other products available which would be just as satisfactory for the purpose.

CONTRAST RADIOGRAPHY OF THE ALIMENTARY TRACT

Indications

This procedure is employed in an attempt to reveal:

1   Obstruction of the alimentary tract by causes such as non-radio-opaque foreign bodies (soft rubber, cloth, etc.), tumour masses or stenosis of the tract.
2   Distortions of the wall of the alimentary tract (oesophageal dilatations, enlargement of the stomach resulting from pyloric stenosis, etc.).
3   Lesions of the wall of the alimentary tract (neoplasia, ulcers, etc.).
4   Displacement of the alimentary tract, either due to the presence of an intra-abdominal mass or in association with a ruptured diaphragm.
5   Normal and abnormal alimentary function.

Contrast agents

A specially prepared fine colloidal suspension of barium sulphate is used routinely for this purpose. It is marketed under a variety of trade names in three different forms (Table 13.1).

1   A ready prepared colloidal suspension, usually containing 100 per cent w/v barium sulphate (e.g. Micropaque Standard or Baritop 100).
2   A fine dry powder which has to be mixed with water to the required consistency prior to use (e.g. Micropaque HD, Baritop G or E-Z-Paque).
3   A thick viscous paste which adhers to mucosa and is used to outline the pharynx and oesophagus ('barium swallow') (e.g. Microtrast).

If there is any possibility that the alimentary tract has been perforated, it might be preferable to use an organic iodine preparation (e.g. Gastro-Conray and Gastrografin, Table 13.2), since any barium that enters a body cavity would not be absorbed or eliminated and could remain *in situ* indefinitely. A water soluble contrast agent, however, would be absorbed from the pleural or peritoneal cavity. Unfortunately, because these agents are hypertonic, they absorb fluid and become diluted, thus producing inferior contrast (see p. 243). The extravasation of fluid can produce hypovolaemic shock in a sick and dehydrated patient. The use of a low osmolar contrast agent would reduce this risk.

Apparatus

A flexible polythene bottle (of 50–100 ml capacity) with a screw-on stopper traversed by a narrow flexible tube, or a large syringe attached to a tube, is of assistance in introducing the watery mixture of barium into the animal's mouth.

A stomach tube can be used with advantage to instil the barium into the stomach more rapidly for upper gastrointestinal examinations.

An enema syringe or gravity feed will be required if the barium is to be administered per rectum.

Preparation of the patient

Prior to the examination the alimentary tract should be emptied by withholding food for some 24 hours, and if necessary, by administering an enema. When dealing with the acutely ill animal there may not be time for such preparation but the tract is likely to have been emptied by vomiting or inappetance. Reduced amounts of barium should be given to an animal which is particularly dehydrated or one which is likely to be subjected to immediate bowel surgery.

The use of general anaesthesia should be avoided as it can slow or arrest the passage of the contrast agent or it may relieve or prevent recognition of any nervous spasm or constriction of the tract. If sedation must be used it should be confined to the phenothiazine derivatives such as acepromazine maleate.

Technique

The barium suspension is usually administered by introducing the nozzle of the bottle or syringe into the side of the dog's mouth and then giving small amounts and allowing time for the dog to swallow before giving more. It is important that the dog should swallow the mixture naturally and that it should not be forcibly squirted down the throat. Otherwise it is only too easy to introduce barium into the trachea. The procedure may take 5–10 minutes and should not be hurried. Unfortunately this usually means that by the time the animal can be positioned for radiography the barium will have left the oesophagus completely and some will have entered the small intestine. To avoid the latter complication, a stomach tube can be used to introduce the barium more rapidly into the stomach. A stomach tube can be passed safely in most cooperative or sedated dogs, but obviously this technique does not permit examination of the oesophagus.

The precise technique employed should be modified in order to facilitate the examination of particular areas of the alimentary tract and these will be described later.

Plain radiographs of the abdomen should be taken in both

Barium enema

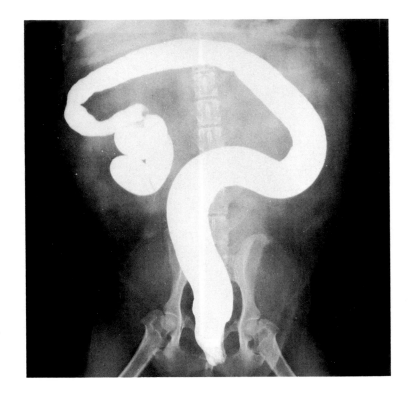

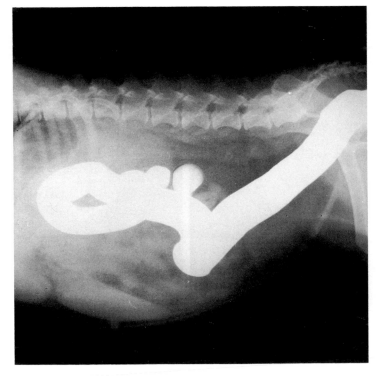

Barium enema

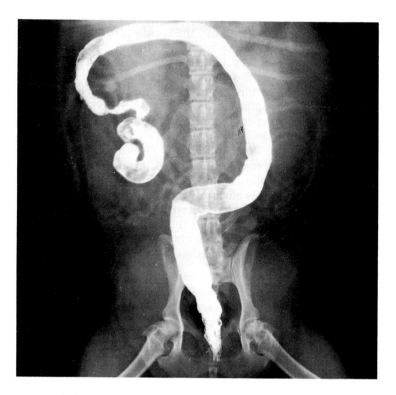

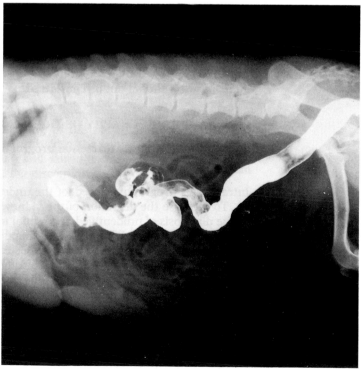

After evacuation.

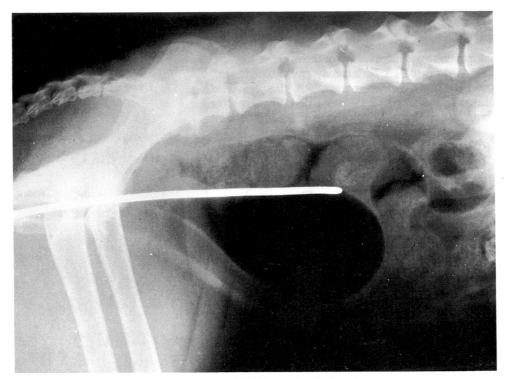

Lateral view of bladder inflated with air.

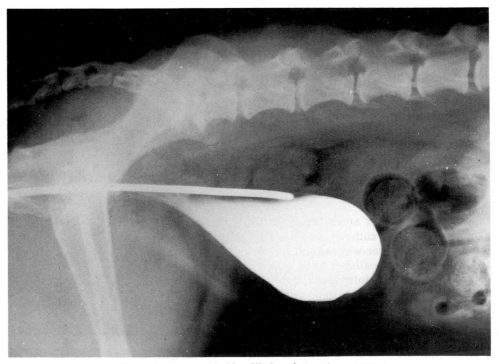

Lateral view of a bladder filled with positive contrast.

there is leakage around the catheter. This technique is cheap and satisfactory for most conditions.

A *positive contrast cystogram* is similar but utilizes water soluble contrast medium to distend the bladder. This technique provides better mucosal detail than the pneumocystogram, but small lesions or calculi may be lost in the contrast pool.

Double contrast cystography provides optimal mucosal detail and is the best method for detecting radiolucent calculi. In this technique, 5 to 15 ml of a water soluble contrast agent are injected into the evacuated bladder, followed by air as for the pneumocystogram. The radiopaque contrast agent coats the mucosa lightly to highlight mucosal or bladder wall lesions and the residual contrast puddle is useful for demonstrating small luminal changes and calculi.

Radiography

The lateral view is usually the most informative but this should be supplemented by a ventrodorsal view and oblique views where indicated.

Close collimation to the caudal abdomen will improve detail. High definition film-screen combinations can be used in all but the larger sized breeds of dog, where a good quality grid should be employed.

Urethrography

Indications

Retrograde urethrography can be used in conjunction with cystography in the following situations:

1   To evaluate the prostate gland in the male.
2   To investigate urinary incontinence (e.g. ureteral ectopia or bladder sphincter mechanism defect).
3   To evaluate the urethra for mucosal defects (e.g. tumours) or for obstruction (e.g. calculi or strictures).
4   To assess displacement or deviation of the urethra (e.g. retroflexion of the bladder).

Contrast agents

Water soluble contrast media containing between 150 and 200 mg iodine per ml (Table 13.2) will provide adequate contrast without irritating the mucosa. If the contrast is mixed with K-Y Jelly (Johnson & Johnson) it will remain in the urethra for a longer period of time which can be of help in this examination.

Apparatus

A dog urinary catheter for the male and a Foley catheter for the bitch are required together with a suitable connector, three-way tap and syringe.

soluble preparations and this has led to the introduction of the low osmolar, non-ionic, water soluble contrast media (Table 13.2) for myelography.

Metrizamide (Amipaque) was the first non-ionic, water soluble contrast medium considered safe enough to be used in veterinary radiology for myelography (Lord and Olsson, 1976; Wright and Clayton Jones, 1981). Metrizamide produces good contrast but side effects occur in a significant number of cases. These include partial or generalized seizures, exacerbation of neurological signs, transient apnoea during injection of the contrast medium and vomiting or hyperaesthesia on recovery. These reactions are usually transient. Deaths have been reported but are considered rare and usually associated with incorrect positioning of the needle. More recently iopamidol (Niopam) and iohexol (Omnipaque) have been introduced. They have fewer side effects than metrizamide and are generally considered to be superior (Wheeler and Davies, 1985). In some cases, iopamidol does not appear to mix with the cerebrospinal fluid and this can cause confusing results. This feature has not been noted with metrizamide or iohexol.

The contrast medium can be introduced into the subarachnoid space following either cisternal or lumbar puncture. The dose depends on the suspected site of the lesion as well as the patient's size. Cervical lesions generally require less contrast than lumbar lesions. A dose rate of 0.3 ml/kg body weight up to a maximum volume of 9 ml should provide an adequate amount of contrast for evaluation of the entire spinal canal. Metrizamide is usually administered as an isotonic solution containing 170 mg iodine per ml, whereas iopamidol and iohexol are usually used at a concentration of 300 mg iodine per ml which is mildly hypertonic. These agents, however, can be diluted to any concentration using saline or cerebrospinal fluid.

Apparatus

A small syringe and a short bevelled spinal or hypodermic needle are required for injecting the contrast medium. A 23 gauge 25 mm (1 inch) needle is usually adequate for cats and small dogs, a 21 gauge 40 mm (1.5 inch) needle for medium-sized dogs and a 21 gauge 75–90 mm (3–3.5 inch) needle for large and giant breeds of dog. It is also necessary to have a surface sloping at about 10–15 degrees on which the patient can be placed to facilitate the passage of the contrast agent along the spinal canal.

Preparation

General anaesthesia is essential and the patient should be intubated in order to maintain an airway, even if gaseous anaesthesia is not used. Acepromazine is best avoided as a premedicant, since it may help induce seizures. Diazepam is considered by many to be a better choice for this investigation. The hair is clipped over the injection site and the skin is aseptically prepared for introduction of the needle.

Technique

The contrast medium is most commonly introduced into the sub-arachnoid space by injection into the cisterna magna. A lumbar puncture, which is technically more difficult to perform, is only necessary when the contrast medium fails to outline the lesion or its caudal flow is insufficient to demonstrate the extent of the lesion. A lumbar puncture can be carried out directly following a cisternal puncture to provide the necessary information when the flow of contrast is obstructed.

Cisternal myelography

The anaesthetized animal is positioned in left lateral recumbency with the head flexed and held by an assistant at approximately 90 degrees to the cervical spine. It is important to check that the airway is not obstructed when the patient is in this position. The radiography table is tilted to 10–15 degrees with the animal's head uppermost. Strict asepsis must be observed during the procedure and thorough disinfection of the skin is essential.

The point of insertion for the needle can be determined from the intersection of two imaginary lines: one in the midline running from the external occipital protruberance to the dorsal spinous process of the axis and the other at right angles to it joining the cranial borders of the wings of the atlas. It is helpful to identify the external occipital protruberance with the middle finger of the left hand while holding the cranial edges of the wings of the atlas between the left thumb and index finger.

The needle is inserted through the skin at the intersection of these lines and directed towards the lower mandible making sure that the needle remains in the midline in order to avoid the cervical venous sinuses which run longitudinally on either side of the midline. The bevel of the needle should be pointing caudally to encourage the flow of contrast down the spine. The needle is advanced slowly. Resistance can be felt as it passes through the ligamentum flavum followed by a 'popping' sensation when it enters the cisterna magna. If the needle strikes bone before it enters the cisterna magna, it should be withdrawn slightly and redirected. Confirmation that the needle has entered the cisterna magna is indicated by clear cerebrospinal fluid dripping from the needle. This occurs spontaneously with a hypodermic needle but only after removal of the stilette with a spinal needle. If blood should appear, the needle should be removed and a fresh puncture made with a new needle.

The cerebrospinal fluid is allowed to drip out until a volume approximately similar to the volume of contrast to be injected has been removed. The fluid can be collected for laboratory analysis if necessary. The syringe containing the contrast medium is attached to the needle and the medium injected slowly over about 2 minutes. Care should be taken to prevent the needle from being pushed further into the animal. If there is any resistance or back pressure, the injection should be terminated and the needle and syringe removed. Occasional aspiration during the injection will show that the needle is still in the subarachnoid space.

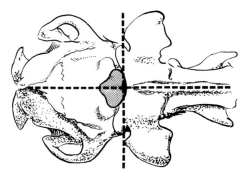

Landmarks for cisternal puncture.

Only one lung can be examined at a time by this method, and where it is necessary to repeat the procedure on the other lung this must be delayed until contrast material has been eliminated from the first lung (usually a delay of 48 hours is necessary).

Selective filling of a single bronchus has been advocated by Bishop, Medway and Archibald (1955) and Zontine (1975). These techniques usually involve the direct introduction of the agent through a catheter positioned in the bronchus under investigation. The placement of the catheter is most easily performed with image intensification. In the authors' experience, however, this does not result in such a good spread of the contrast medium.

CHOLECYSTOGRAPHY

Indications

Indications for this technique are limited. The main purpose of this procedure is to demonstrate the main bile ducts and gall-bladder in the investigation of a ruptured bile duct, suspected calculi or other lesions of the area; conditions which are rare in small animals. It has been suggested that observation of the excretion of the contrast agent provides a means of assessing liver function. However, this can probably be more accurately assessed by biochemical means. The procedure should be used with caution in cases of severe liver damage since it is unlikely that much of the contrast will be excreted via the biliary system, although in most instances the agent will then be excreted by the kidneys.

Contrast agents

The most satisfactory products are those for intravenous use given either by injection or infusion (Table 13.3). These water soluble iodine compounds are protein bound in the circulation and very largely excreted through the biliary system. The preparations for intravenous injection (Biliscopin and Biligram) contain approximately 180 mg iodine per ml in a 30 per cent solution and should be administered at a dose rate of 0.5 ml per kg body weight. Intravenous injection in the conscious patient may cause some discomfort—the dog moves uneasily and may retch or vomit. These side effects are reduced by slow intravenous infusion of the contrast agent (Biliscopin or Biligram for infusion). These preparations contain between 50 and 85 mg iodine per ml and should be given at a dose rate of 1.0 ml per kg body weight, the total dose being infused over about 30 minutes.

Oral preparations are used in man (Biloptin and Telepaque) but these have proved less satisfactory in the dog, since absorption is variable.

Apparatus

This comprises an intravenous needle or catheter and a syringe or infusion set suitable for administration of the contrast agent.

Preparation of the patient

Food and water should be withheld for 12 hours prior to the injection of the contrast agent.

General anaesthesia may be employed in order to avoid the patient feeling any discomfort and to prevent movement during radiography, but this would have to be maintained for some 2 hours and would interfere with subsequent feeding of the dog to provoke emptying of the gallbladder.

Technique

The contrast agent is administered either by slow intravenous injection over about 3 minutes or by infusion over about 30 minutes. Once the gallbladder has been satisfactorily outlined a small, preferably fatty, meal may be given to demonstrate adequate emptying of the gallbladder.

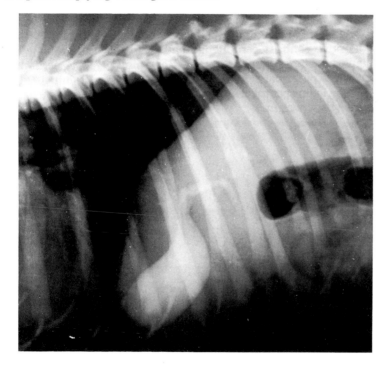

Cholecystogram 90 minutes after injection of contrast medium.

Radiography

A lateral radiograph of the cranial abdomen centring over the liver, is the most informative view. Close collimation to the area of interest will improve definition and if the depth of soft tissue is greater than 10 to 15 cm, a good quality grid should also be employed. The lateral view can be supplemented by one taken in the ventrodorsal plane (this view is not so useful because the caudal border of the lungs will be superimposed on the liver and gall bladder shadow). Radiographs are taken immediately before injection of the drug and 20 to 30 minutes (when the bile ducts are most satisfactorily demonstrated) and 90 minutes (for maximum concentration of contrast agent within the gallbladder) after administration. Final radiographs will be taken some 15 minutes after the meal given to provoke emptying of the gallbladder.

Dorn, A. S. (1972) A standard technique for canine cerebral angiography. *J. Am. vet. med. Ass.*, **161**, 12.

Ettinger, S. J. & Suter, P. F. (1970) Cardiac catheterization and angiocardiography. In: *Canine Cardiology*, p. 170. Philadelphia: W. B. Saunders.

Evans, S. M. & Laufer, I. (1981) Double contrast gastrography in the normal dog. *Vet. Radiol.*, **22**, 2.

Gelatt, K. N., Cure, T. H., Guffy, M. H. & Jessen, C. (1972) Dacrocystorhinography in the dog and cat. *J. small Anim. Pract.*, **13**, 381.

Hamlin, R. (1959) Angiocardiography for the clinical diagnosis of congenital heart disease in small animals. *J. Am. vet. med. Ass.*, **135**, 112.

Harvey, C. E. (1969) Sialography in the dog. *J. Am. vet. Radiol. Soc.*, **10**, 18.

Holt, P. E., Gibbs, C. & Pearson, H. (1982) Canine ectopic ureter—a review of twenty nine cases. *J. small Anim. Pract.*, **23**, 195.

Holt, P. E., Gibbs, C. & Latham, J. (1984) An evaluation of positive contrast vagino-urethrography as a diagnostic aid in the bitch. *J. small Anim. Pract.*, **25**, 531.

James, C. W. & Hoerlein, B.F. (1960) Cerebral angiography in the dog. *Vet. Med.*, **55**, 45.

Lee, R. & Griffiths, I. R. (1972) A comparison of cerebral arteriography and cavernous sinus venography in the dog. *J. small Anim. Pract.*, **13**, 225.

Lord, P. F., Scott, R. C. & Chan, K. F. (1974) Intravenous urography for evaluation of renal diseases in small animals. *J. Am. Anim. Hosp. Ass.*, **10**, 139.

Lord, P. F. & Olsson, S-E. (1976) Myelography with metrizamide in the dog: a clinical study on its use for the demonstration of spinal cord lesions other than those caused by intervertebral disc protrusion. *J. Am. vet. Radiol. Soc.*, **17**, 42.

Oliver, J. E., Jr. (1969) Cranial sinus venography in the dog. *J. Am. vet. Radiol. Soc.*, **10**, 66.

Owen, L. N. & Hall, L. W. (1962) Ascites in a dog due to a metastasis from an adenocarcinoma of the ovary. *Vet. Rec.*, **74**, 220.

Prier, J. E., Schaffer, B. & Skelley, J. F. (1962) Direct lymphangiography in the dog. *J. Am. vet. med. Ass.*, **140**, 943.

Rendano, V. T. (1979) Positive contrast peritoneography: An aid in the radiographic diagnosis of diaphragmatic hernia. *J. Am. vet. Radiol. Soc.*, **20**, 67.

Root, C. R. & Morgan, J. P. (1969) Contrast radiography of the upper gastrointestinal tract in the dog. *J. small Anim. Pract.*, **10**, 279.

Suter, P. F. & Carb, A. V. (1969) Shoulder arthrography in dogs—radiographic anatomy and clinical application. *J. small Anim. Pract.*, **10**, 407.

Suter, P. F. (1975) Portal vein anomalies in the dog: their angiographic diagnosis. *J. Am. vet. Radiol. Soc.*, **16**, 84.

Suter, P. F. (1983) Diseases of the peripheral vessels. In: *Textbook of Veterinary Internal Medicine* (ed. S. J. Ettinger), 2nd edn., p. 1062. Philadelphia: W. B. Saunders.

Wheeler, S. J. & Davies, J. V. (1985) Iohexol myelography in the dog and cat: a series of one hundred cases, and a comparison with metrizamide and iopamidol. *J. small Anim. Pract.*, **26**, 247.

Wright, J. A. & Clayton Jones, D. G. (1981) Metrizamide myelography in sixty-eight dogs. *J. small Anim. Pract.*, **22**, 415.

Zontine, W. J. (1975) Bronchography in the dog. In: *Radiographic Technique in Small Animal Practice* (ed. J. W. Ticer), p. 315. Philadelphia: W. B. Saunders.

INTRODUCTION

Radiography of the horse poses problems with regard to the thickness of the tissue to be penetrated, restraint and additional risks to assistants holding the animal or the film. These difficulties must be considered in some detail under four headings.

Size of patient

While young foals and a few miniature ponies correspond in size to the larger breeds of dog and can be positioned and radiographed similarly, radiography of the majority of horses will require penetration of a much denser area of tissue. This involves much greater output of the X-ray apparatus and, in the case of the smaller machines, can be obtained only by increasing the exposure time, which in turn involves a risk of blurring from movement unless the horse can be adequately restrained by anaesthetization and casting. Thus the extent of the radiography which can be undertaken on the standing horse will be governed very largely by the power of the apparatus available. The diagram below gives some idea of which parts may be penetrated with different types of machine in a horse of 540–680 kg (1200–1500 lb) weight.

The scope of each type of apparatus can be considerably extended if the animal can be anaesthetized and restrained for relatively long periods.

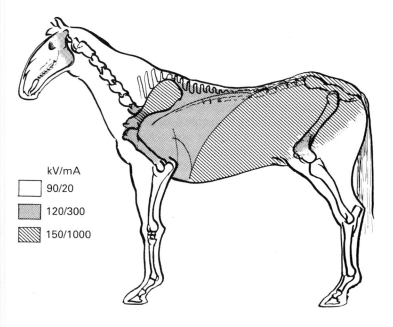

kV/mA

☐ 90/20

▨ 120/300

▧ 150/1000

Restraint

Most equine radiography is undertaken with the horse standing and therefore comparatively unrestrained. For this reason the procedure is always time-consuming and should be carefully thought out and planned before commencing the examination.

For the benefit of radiographers with little experience of this

2 Distal Sesamoid (Navicular) Bone

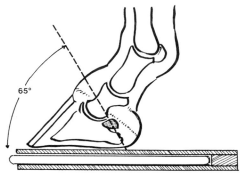

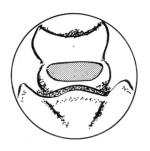

DORSOPROXIMAL–PALMARODISTAL OBLIQUE (DORSOPALMAR OR HIGH CORONARY VIEW)

The horse stands on a cassette tunnel (see p.126) containing a cassette. It is helpful if the cassette tunnel is marked to show the correct position for the foot in order to project the navicular bone in the centre of the film.

The central ray is directed down through the navicular bone at an angle of about 65° from the horizontal and centred just above the coronary band.

Tight collimation and the use of high definition film–screen combinations will enhance detail. If only regular film–screen combinations are available then a good-quality grid should be employed, but this must be protected from pressure damage.

DORSOPROXIMAL–PLANTARODISTAL OBLIQUE (DORSOPLANTAR)

This view is essentially the same. However outward rotation of the leg is advised in order to prevent placing the tube under the horse.

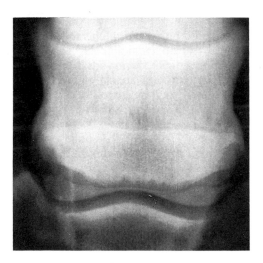

Exposure factors					
	kV	mA	Sec	Grid	Notes
Average pony					
Average hunter					

Film type: Screen type: FFD:

PALMAROPROXIMAL–PALMARODISTAL OBLIQUE (FLEXOR SURFACE)

This view can only be taken in the very quiet or sedated horse, since the tube is placed immediately behind the limb. The foot is positioned on a cassette tunnel containing a cassette. The beam is angled to about 65° and centred to the midpoint between the bulbs of the heel. The angulation should be as steep as possible without producing superimposition of the fetlock. The precise angle will vary with the conformation of the horse. In order to position the tube head, it is necessary to reduce the focal–film distance.

PLANTAROPROXIMAL–PLANTARODISTAL OBLIQUE

This view is essentially the same.

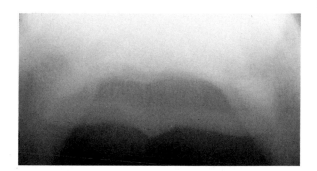

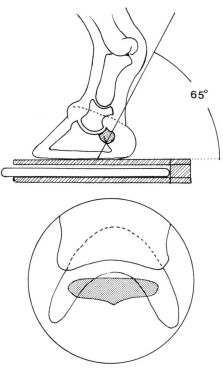

2 Distal Sesamoid (Navicular) Bone

65°

Exposure factors					
	kV	mA	Sec	Grid	Notes
Average pony					
Average hunter					

Film type: Screen type: FFD:

LATERAL

A lateral view of the navicular bone can be taken using the positioning for the distal phalanx (see p. 295). Centre along the navicular bone which lies approximately halfway between the coronet and sole and two-thirds caudally along the hoof. To ensure a true lateral projection, check that the beam is parallel to a line across the bulbs of the heels. Exposure factors can be based on those for the lateral view of the pedal bone (p. 295).

4 Metacarpophalangeal or Metatarsophalangeal (Fetlock) Joint

DORSOPALMAR OR DORSOPLANTAR (ANTEROPOSTERIOR)

The animal stands normally. The cassette in a holder is placed immediately behind the joint and angled slightly to permit demonstration of the joint space. The central ray is directed through the joint at right-angles to the film.

The sesamoid bones

The mA-s factor should be doubled for improved visualization of the proximal sesamoid bones.

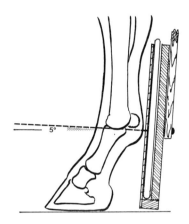

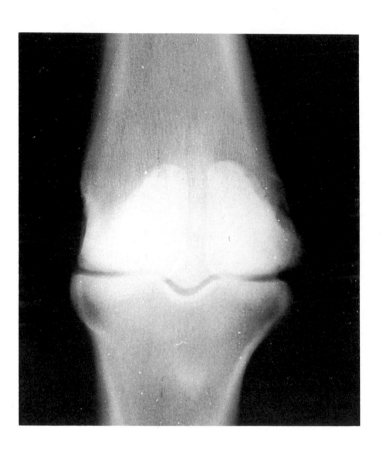

Exposure factors					
	kV	mA	Sec	Grid	Notes
Average pony					
Average hunter					

Film type: Screen type: FFD:

LATERAL

The cassette in a holder is placed against the medial aspect of the limb. The central ray is directed horizontally through the joint, at right-angles to the film.

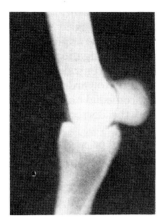

FLEXED LATERAL

The limb under investigation is raised and the fetlock flexed. The cassette in a holder is placed against the medial aspect of the joint and the beam centred horizontally through the joint. Since it is necessary to hold the limb for this projection, close collimation and adequate protection are essential.

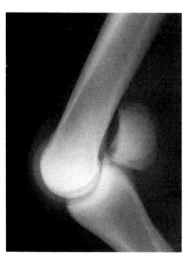

4 Metacarpo-phalangeal or Metatarsophalangeal (Fetlock) Joint

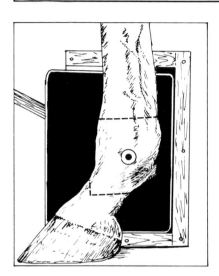

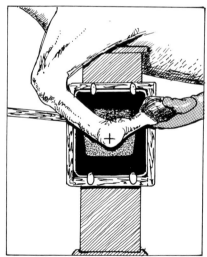

Exposure factors					
	kV	mA	Sec	Grid	Notes
Average pony					
Average hunter					

Film type: Screen type: FFD:

6 Carpus

DORSOLATERAL–PALMAROMEDIAL OBLIQUE
DORSOMEDIAL–PALMAROLATERAL OBLIQUE

Oblique views are essential for the full investigation of the carpus and are necessary for demonstrating small exostoses or chip fractures, since these may not be seen on the standard projections. The beam is angled approximately 45° from the dorsal midline centring through the midpoint of the carpus. The cassette holder must be securely supported.

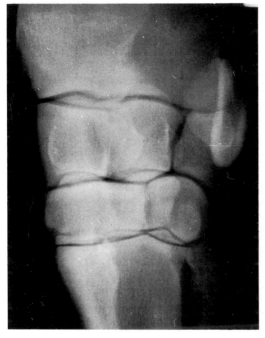

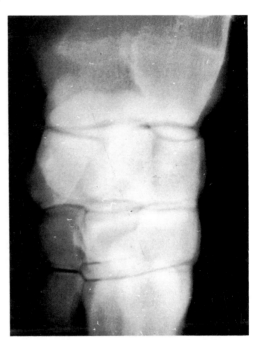

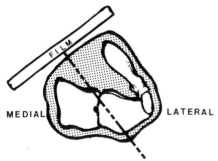

Dorsolateral–palmaromedial oblique

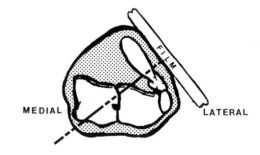

Dorsomedial–palmarolateral oblique

Exposure factors					
	kV	mA	Sec	Grid	Notes
Average pony					
Average hunter					

Film type: Screen type: FFD:

DORSOPROXIMAL–DORSODISTAL OBLIQUE (SKYLINE)

With the carpus flexed, the beam is directed down on to the dorsal surface of the carpus in order to highlight the proximal row of carpal bones (A) or the distal row (B). The cassette in a holder is placed in line with the metacarpus and parallel to the floor.

6 Carpus

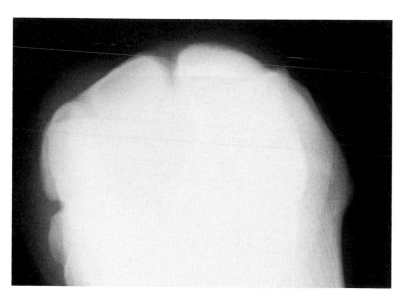

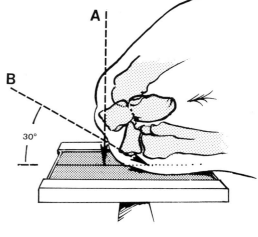

Exposure factors						
	kV	mA	Sec	Grid	Notes	
Average pony						
Average hunter						

Film type: Screen type: FFD:

Chapter 15

Other Species

The importance of veterinary radiography as a diagnostic tool is shown by the fact that it has now been used in the investigation of problems involving a very large number of domesticated and wild creatures varying from insects to elephants. Obviously, however, it is not possible, within the scope of this book, to attempt to list and describe the many examinations which the veterinary radiographer may wish to attempt in other species of animal. Fortunately in most instances he will find that he can employ positioning and exposure factors similar to, or deduced from, those described for the dog and the horse.

In this chapter, therefore, the authors have confined themselves to commenting generally on some of the problems likely to be encountered with other types of patient and to drawing attention to certain specialized examinations which are now being undertaken in some domestic animals. Inevitably there will be many omissions, but in the authors' experience, provided that the patient can be adequately restrained, there should be no problem for the experienced radiographer in adapting a radiographic technique suitable for one type of animal to a completely new species.

FARM ANIMALS

The extent to which radiography is employed in the investigation of farm animals will be influenced by a number of considerations:

1 Economic factors will always restrict the extent to which potentially costly diagnostic procedures or even treatments can be employed for farm animals. However, with the advent of more efficient apparatus and techniques, radiography is being employed to an ever increasing extent in the examination of the more valuable farm animals.
2 The practicability of restraining the animal (this will often necessitate the induction of general anaesthesia) or of transporting it to where suitable high power apparatus is available.
3 The availability of suitable X-ray machines and accessory equipment. Only a limited number of X-ray examinations can be carried out with portable apparatus on the farm and many investigations require the animal to be transported to a site where more powerful and suitable equipment is available. The diagrams of the ox, sheep and pig (pp. 335, 339 and 340 respectively) have been compiled to correspond with that of the horse on p. 287 and are intended to give some indication of the radiographic output necessary for the investigation of various parts of these animals. The three differently shaded areas demonstrate those parts which may be penetrated by portable, mobile, or fixed high output X-ray apparatus. This is a rather arbitrary division and, in practice, it will be affected by a number of factors:

 a The actual size of the animal being examined. There is obviously a great difference between the radiographic output necessary to penetrate the lumbar region of a thin dairy heifer and that required for the same area of a large, fully mature bull.
 b The precise output of the X-ray apparatus to be used. There is a wide variation in the power of machines of the 'mobile'

group and those with lower output are not suitable for penetrating the denser parts.

c The skill of the radiographer and the ancillary apparatus available. The use of rare-earth screens will increase the scope of the examinations which can be undertaken with lower power machines. Similarly, a grid with a high ratio is required to control scatter when X-raying particularly thick areas of tissue (e.g. the spine of a bull) but this can only be used effectively if some means of aligning the primary beam accurately with the grid is also available (see p. 127).

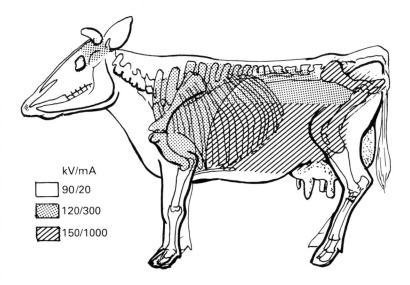

kV/mA
☐ 90/20
▨ 120/300
▨ 150/1000

THE OX

The distal limb

Radiography of the lower limbs is possible in the standing animal using positioning similar to that advocated for the horse (pp. 291–314).

Further comment is given concerning the examination of the foot as this is the region most frequently radiographed in this species.

tapes can do. If more than one exposure is to be made, it is preferable to fix the bird to a piece of film cardboard or 2 mm thick 'Perspex' sheet.

Whole body views in both planes should be taken of small birds. In both the ventrodorsal and lateral projections, the wings and legs must be fully extended and secured. To prevent superimposition in the lateral view, the appendages nearest to the film are extended cranially and contralateral limbs caudally, and identified with markers.

Larger birds may require special views of the appendicular skeleton but the principles of restraint outlined above still apply.

Care should be taken to keep small, shocked birds warm during the examination.

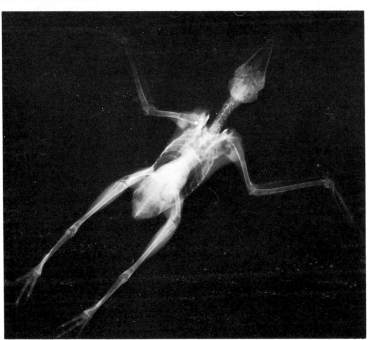

A ventrodorsal view of a rook.

Exposure factors				
	kV	mA	Sec	Notes

Film type: Screen type: FFD:

SMALL PETS AND LABORATORY ANIMALS

Rats, mice, rabbits, ferrets and other small animals which are kept as pets or for laboratory purposes may be radiographed as individuals for the investigation of traumatic or other disease processes.

The small size of the majority of these animals causes problems, as they are difficult to position without recourse to sedation or anaesthesia and the laboratory method of placing them in a plastic tube results in a film in which neither limbs or body are properly visualized. Using the methods of anaesthesia described by Jones

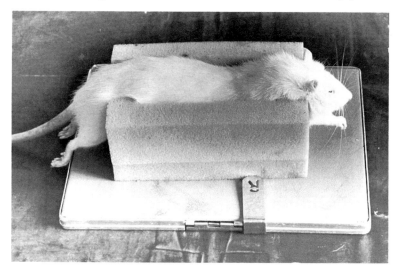

(1977) and Cooper *et al* (1985) the animals can be positioned in a similar manner to that described for birds by fixing them on to the film with masking tape.

When anaesthesia is contraindicated, it is helpful to make a cradle out of polyfoam or polystyrene. This not only restrains the small wriggling creature but is warm and soothing. A fast exposure time will be necessary in case there is still some movement.

Long-term studies

The veterinary radiographer may also be asked to undertake the monitoring of a group of laboratory animals which are being kept to assess the long-term effects of the administration of a particular drug or treatment. This is likely to involve repeated radiography, at regular intervals, of a particular organ (usually a bone or joint) under exactly comparable conditions.

When such a long-term investigation is contemplated it is important that there should be very careful preparation, and even a pilot experiment, before embarking on the project. The radiographer should always consider the following points:

1 *Positioning* Very heavy sedation or general anaesthesia is mandatory as the animals must be placed in positions which can be repeated precisely. They must never be held by hand and it is

PRIMATES

This group of animals poses problems with regard to both human health hazards and the difficulty of restraining the patient. Handling of primates should therefore always be undertaken by their usual attendants and not by inexperienced volunteers.

Animals of this group vary considerably in size but, provided they can be anaesthetized or heavily sedated, exposure factors selected from those for dogs of equivalent weight and thickness should prove suitable.

Particular problems may however be encountered when X-raying the thorax, an area which is frequently examined, either for the routine screening of imported animals, or for subsequent research purposes. Bear in mind that, in contrast to most other animals, the chest of this species is thinnest in the ventrodorsal direction and that this projection will provide the most informative visualization of the thorax. This view is usually employed in preference to the dorsoventral projection because, when sedated,

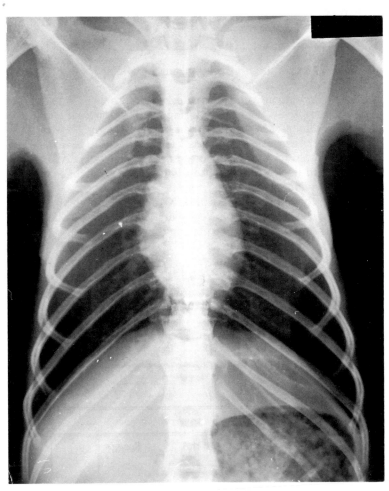

A dorsoventral view of the lungs of an adult Rhesus monkey.

primates tend to adopt a crouching position and are then difficult to position dorsoventrally.

Another difficulty associated with thoracic radiography of primates is that they vary considerably in the size and conformation of this area and three examples will be given to illustrate this.

The common marmoset (*Callithrix jacchus*) is small, very fine boned and has no excessive musculature. The depth of the chest is about 4 cm thick and the diaphragm is surprisingly low. It is very easy therefore to overexpose the lung fields and to prevent this the use of high definition films and screens are advised.

The Rhesus monkey (*Macaca mulatta*) is larger, weighing between 5 and 10 kilograms, but does not show any unusual conformation and radiography is reasonably straightforward.

The stumptailed macaque (*Macaca arctoides*), which weighs about 15 kilograms when adult, has a high diaphragm and a relatively thick muscle layer which overlies the thorax. This musculature makes it imperative to use a grid when X-raying the lung fields in order to achieve reasonable contrast.

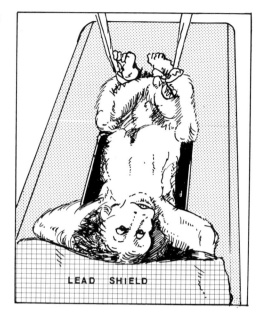

LEAD SHIELD

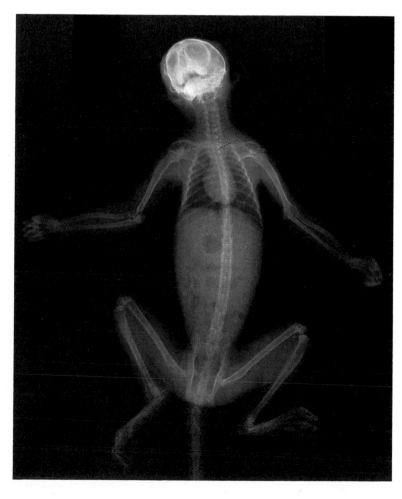

A whole body view of the common marmoset.

It must be stressed that members of this group do show considerable differences from the usual veterinary patients and that radiographers who are likely to be required to examine them frequently would be well advised to consult those with experience in this field (Silverman and Hoffman, 1973) or to refer to the positioning and exposure factors advised for children.

Exposure factors				
	kV	mA	Sec	Notes

Film type: Screen type: FFD:

REFERENCES

Ardran, G. H. and Brown, T. H. (1964) X-ray diagnosis of pregnancy in sheep with special reference to the determination of the number of foetuses. *J. agric. Sci., Camb.*, **63**, 205.

Cooper, J. E., Hutchison, M. F., Jackson, O. F. and Maurice, R. J. (1985) *Manual of Exotic Pets*, Cheltenham, Glos., B.S.A.V.A.

Done, J. T. (1976) Porcine atrophic rhinitis: snout radiography as an aid to diagnosis and detection of the disease. *Vet. Rec.*, **98**, 23.

Jones, D. M. (1977) The sedation and anaesthesia of birds and reptiles. *Vet. Rec.*, **101**, 340.

Silverman, S. and Hoffman, R. (1972–73) The restraint apparatus of exotic animals and birds. *Am. Ass. Zoo Vets ann. Proc.*, 174.

PHYSICS

Curry, T. S., Dowdey, J. E. and Murry, R. C. (1984) *Christensen's Introduction to the Physics of Diagnostic Radiology*. Philadelphia: Lea and Febiger.

Gifford, D. (1984) *A Handbook of Physics for Radiologists and Radiographers*. Chichester: John Wiley and Sons.

Hay, G. A. and Hughes, D. (1983) *First-Year Physics for Radiographers*, 3rd edn. London: Baillière Tindall.

Meredith, W. J. and Massey, J. B. (1977) *Fundamental Physics of Radiology*, 3rd edn. Bristol: John Wright and Sons.

RADIATION HAZARDS AND PROTECTION

Health and Safety Commission (1985) Approved Code of Practice. The Protection of Persons Against Ionising Radiation Arising from any Work Activity. The Ionising Radiation Regulations 1985. London: HMSO.

Health and Safety Executive (1986) Guidance Notes for the Protection of Persons Against Ionising Radiations Arising from Veterinary Use. London: HMSO (in preparation).

Lee, R. (1978) Radiation in veterinary practice. *Vet. Rec. 103*, 97–100.

O'Riordan, M. C. (1970) Examination of a veterinary practice for radiation hazards. *J. small Anim. Pract. 11*, 515–522.

Unwin, D. D. (1970) Radiation protection in veterinary practice. *J small Anim. Pract. 11*, 523–532.

VETERINARY RADIOGRAPHY AND RADIOLOGY

Douglas, S. W. and Williamson, H. D. (1970) Veterinary Radiological Interpretation. London: Heinemann Veterinary Books.

Felson, B. (Ed.) (1968) *Roentgen Techniques in Laboratory Animals*. Philadelphia: W. B. Saunders.

Gillette, E. L., Thrall, D. E. and Lebel, J. L. (1977) *Carlson's Veterinary Radiology*, 3rd edn. Philadelphia: Lea and Febiger.

Kealy, J. K. (1986) *Diagnostic Radiology of the Dog and Cat*, 2nd edn. Philadelphia: W. B. Saunders.

Kealy, J. K. (Ed.) (1982) Symposium on radiology. *Vet. Clin. N. Am.*, 12, 2.

Kleine, L. J. (1983) *Small Animal Radiography*. St Louis: Mosby.

Morgan, J. P. (1972) *Radiology in Veterinary Orthopaedics*. Philadelphia: Lea and Febiger.

Morgan, J. P. and Silverman, S. (1982) *Techniques in Veterinary Radiography*, 3rd edn. Davis, Calif.: Veterinary Radiology Associates.

O'Brien, T. R. (1978) *Radiographic Diagnosis of Abdominal Disorders in the Dog and Cat*. Philadelphia: W. B. Saunders.

Olsson, S.-E. (1973) *Radiological Diagnosis in Canine and Feline Emergencies*. Philadelphia: Lea and Febiger.

Ryan, G. D. (1981) *Radiographic Positioning of Small Animals*. Philadelphia: Lea and Febiger.

Schebitz, H. and Wilkens, H. (1986) *Atlas of Radiographic Anatomy of Dog, Cat and Horse*, 4th edn., vols 1 and 2. Berlin: Paul Parey.

Smallwood, J. E., Shively, M. J., Rendano, V. T. and Habel, R. E. (1985) A standardized nomenclature for the radiographic projections used in veterinary medicine. *Vet. Radiol.*, 26, 2–9.

Suter, P. F. (Ed.) (1974) Symposium on radiology. *Vet. Clin. N. Am.*, 4, 4.

Suter, P. F. (1984) *Thoracic Radiography of the Dog and Cat.* Wettswil, Switzerland: P. F. Suter.

Thrall, D. E. (1986) *Textbook of Veterinary Diagnostic Radiology.* Philadelphia: W. B. Saunders.

Ticer, J. W. (1984) *Radiographic Techniques in Small Animal Practice,* 2nd edn. Philadelphia: W. B. Saunders.

Webbon, P. M. (Ed.) (1981) *A Guide to Diagnostic Radiography in Small Animal Practice.* London: B.S.A.V.A.

The following series of articles provide some useful information about radiographic techniques in the horse:

Burguez, P. N. (1984) Interpreting radiographs 4: The carpus. *Equine vet. J. 16,* 159.

Colles, C. M. (1983) Interpreting radiographs 1: The foot. *Equine vet. J. 15,* 297.

Dyson, S. (1986) Interpreting radiographs 7: Radiology of the equine shoulder and elbow. *Equine vet. J. 18,* 352.

Edwards, G. B. (1984) Interpreting radiographs 2: The fetlock joint and pastern. *Equine vet. J. 16,* 4.

Jeffcott, L. B. (1984) Interpreting radiographs 3: Radiology of the stifle joint of the horse. *Equine vet. J. 16,* 81.

Shelley, J. & Dyson, S. (1984) Interpreting radiographs 5: Radiology of the equine hock. *Equine vet. J. 16,* 488.

Wyn-Jones, G. (1985) Interpreting radiographs 6: The head. *Equine vet. J. 17,* 274.

Wyn-Jones, G. (1985) Interpreting radiographs 6: Radiology of the equine head (Part 2). *Equine vet. J. 17,* 417.

Other articles of radiographic interest may be found in journals such as *Veterinary Radiology* and the *Journal of Small Animal Practice.*

DEAN 120 kV 300 mA 4-VALVE MOBILE UNIT

Small animal

Standard screens.
Medium-speed film.
1 metre focal–film distance.
8:1 grid used where indicated. Apparatus operated at 300 mA.

Position no.	Part	View	5 kg		20 kg		40 kg	
			kV	sec	kV	sec	kV	sec
Forelimb								
1	Scapula	CdCr	60	0.04	65	0.10 Grid	70	0.20 Grid
		Lat	60	0.02	70	0.02	70	0.04
2	Shoulder	Lat	48	0.02	60	0.02	62	0.06
3	Humerus	CrCd	52	0.04	60	0.02	65	0.04
		CdCr	52	0.04	60	0.02	65	0.04
		Lat.	48	0.02	55	0.02	62	0.02
4	Elbow	CrCd	50	0.04	57	0.02	60	0.02
		Lat.	48	0.02	55	0.02	57	0.02
5	Radius and ulna	CrCd	45	0.02	50	0.02	55	0.02
		Lat.	45	0.02	50	0.02	55	0.02
6	Carpus	DPa	45	0.02	50	0.02	55	0.02
		Obl.	45	0.02	50	0.02	55	0.02
		Lat.	45	0.02	50	0.02	57	0.02
7	Metacarpus	DPa	45	0.02	50	0.02	55	0.02
		Lat.	45	0.02	52	0.02	57	0.02
8	Digits	DPa	40	0.02	40	0.02	45	0.02
		Lat.	35	0.02	40	0.02	42	0.02
Hindlimb								
10	Hip joint	VD	52	0.04	65	0.04	70	0.04
	Through pelvis	Lat.	60	0.04	65	0.06	72	0.06
	Through joint	Lat.	55	0.04	60	0.02	65	0.04
11	Femur	CrCd	52	0.04	65	0.04	70	0.04
		Lat.	50	0.02	57	0.02	65	0.04
	Through body	Lat.	60	0.02	67	0.04	80	0.10**Grid
12	Stifle	CrCd	55	0.02	65	0.04	70	0.02
		Lat.	50	0.02	57	0.02	65	0.02
	Trochlear gr.		45	0.02	50	0.02	55	0.02
13	Tibia and fibula	CrCd	55	0.02	65	0.02	65	0.02
		Lat.	50	0.02	55	0.02	60	0.02
14	Tarsus	DPl	45	0.02	57	0.02	60	0.02
		Lat.	45	0.02	55	0.02	60	0.02
15	Metatarsus	DPl	45	0.02	55	0.02	60	0.02
		Lat.	45	0.02	57	0.02	62	0.02

** *Apparatus operated at 200 mA.*

DEAN 120 kV 300 mA 4-VALVE MOBILE UNIT

Small animal

Standard screens.
Medium-speed film.
1 metre focal–film distance.
8:1 grid used where indicated. Apparatus operated at 300 mA.

Position no.	Part	View	5 kg		20 kg		40 kg	
			kV	sec	kV	sec	kV	sec
Skull								
16	General	DV	45	0.02	57	0.02	62	0.02
		VD	60	0.02	65	0.04	75	0.08
		Lat.	60	0.02	65	0.04	75	0.08
17	Cranium and	RCd	62	0.02	67	0.04	75	0.10
	sinuses	VD	62	0.02	67	0.04	75	0.08
19	Nasal chambers	VD	50	0.02	60	0.04	65	0.02
20	Temporo-	Lat.	60	0.02	67	0.04	75	0.08
	mandibular joints	Obl.	60	0.02	67	0.04	75	0.08
	Teeth							
22	Upper incisors	IO*	40	0.02‡	45	0.02‡	50	0.02‡
	Upper molars	Obl	50	0.02	50	0.02	55	0.02
	Upper molars	Open mouth	40	0.02	45	0.02	50	0.02
23	Lower incisors	IO*	45	0.02‡	50	0.02‡	55	0.02‡
	Lower molars	Open mouth	40	0.02	45	0.02	50	0.02
	Lower molars	Occ.†	60	0.06‡	65	0.06‡	70	0.06‡
Spine								
25	Cervical	VD	60	0.04	65	0.04	70	0.08 Grid
		Lat.	60	0.04	65	0.04	70	0.04
26	Cervico-	VD	65	0.04	70	0.04	80	0.15**Grid
	thoracic	Lat.	60	0.04	67	0.06	75	0.08 Grid
27	Thoracic	VD	62	0.04	75	0.06	75	0.15 Grid
		Lat.	62	0.02	65	0.04	75	0.06
28	Thoraco-lumbar	VD	62	0.04	75	0.06	75	0.15 Grid
		Lat.	60	0.04	65	0.06	75	0.10 Grid
29	Sacrum	VD	60	0.04	67	0.06	75	0.10 Grid
		Lat.	62	0.04	67	0.06	80	0.10**Grid
30	Coccyx	DV	45	0.02	60	0.02	60	0.02
		Lat.	45	0.02	60	0.02	60	0.02
Soft tissue								
2	Pharynx	Lat.	58	0.02	70	0.02	75	0.06
3	Lungs	DV	65	0.02	75	0.04	90	0.04** Grid
		Lat.	60	0.02	70	0.02	75	0.04
4	Abdomen	VD	60	0.04	75	0.06	100	0.10** Grid
		Lat.	60	0.02	67	0.04	80	0.10** Grid

* *Kodak Non-screen film.*
† *Kodak Fast Occlusal film.*
** *Apparatus operated at 200 mA.*
‡ *30 cm focal–film distance.*

DEAN 120 kV 300 mA 4-VALVE MOBILE UNIT

Average equine (not distal limb)

Standard screens.
Medium-speed film.
1 metre focal–film distance.
8:1 grid used where indicated.

Position no.	Part	View	kV	sec	mA
3	Shoulder	Obl./Lat.	100	0.40	200 Grid
10	Elbow	CrCd	85	0.25	200 Grid
		Lat.	65	0.06	300
16	Skull	VD	95	0.15	200
		R lat.	70	0.12	300
		Cd lat.	80	0.25	200 Grid
		Obl.	60	0.06	300
	Spine				
18	Cervical spine	Lat.	80	0.25	200 Grid
19	Thoracic processes	Lat.	65	0.06	300

A.E.I. (NEWTON-VICTOR) K.5 (G.E. F.4) 15 mA PORTABLE UNIT

Small animal

Standard screens.
Medium-speed film.
75 cm focal–film distance.
Apparatus operated at 15 mA.

Position No.	Part	View	5 kg Stud	5 kg sec	20 kg Stud	20 kg sec	40 kg Stud	40 kg sec
Forelimb								
1	Scapula	CdCr	1	$\frac{1}{4}$	2	$\frac{3}{8}$	3	$\frac{1}{2}$–$\frac{3}{4}$
		Lat.	1	$\frac{1}{8}$	1	$\frac{3}{16}$	3	$\frac{3}{16}$
2	Shoulder	Lat.	1	$\frac{1}{8}$	1	$\frac{3}{16}$	2	$\frac{3}{16}$
3	Humerus	CrCd	1	$\frac{1}{8}$	2	$\frac{1}{4}$	3	$\frac{1}{4}$
		CdCr	1	$\frac{1}{8}$	2	$\frac{1}{8}$	3	$\frac{1}{4}$
		Lat.	1	$\frac{1}{8}$	1	$\frac{3}{16}$	2	$\frac{3}{16}$
4	Elbow	CrCd	1	$\frac{1}{8}$	1	$\frac{1}{4}$	2	$\frac{1}{4}$
		Lat.	1	$\frac{1}{8}$	1	$\frac{3}{16}$	2	$\frac{3}{16}$
5	Radius and ulna	CrCd	1	$\frac{1}{8}$	1	$\frac{3}{16}$	2	$\frac{3}{16}$
		Lat.	1	$\frac{1}{8}$	1	$\frac{1}{8}$	2	$\frac{1}{8}$
6	Carpus	DPa	1	$\frac{1}{8}$	1	$\frac{1}{8}$	2	$\frac{3}{16}$
		Obl.	1	$\frac{1}{8}$	1	$\frac{1}{8}$	2	$\frac{3}{16}$
		Lat.	1	$\frac{1}{8}$	1	$\frac{3}{16}$	2	$\frac{1}{4}$
7	Metacarpus	DPa	1	$\frac{1}{8}$	1	$\frac{1}{8}$	1	$\frac{1}{4}$
		Lat.	1	$\frac{1}{8}$	2	$\frac{1}{8}$	2	$\frac{1}{4}$
8	Digits	DPa	1	$\frac{1}{8}$*	1	$\frac{1}{8}$*	1	$\frac{1}{8}$*
		Lat.	1	$\frac{1}{8}$*	1	$\frac{1}{8}$*	1	$\frac{1}{8}$*
Hindlimb								
10	Hip joint	VD	1	$\frac{1}{8}$	2	$\frac{1}{4}$	3	$\frac{1}{2}$
	Through pelvis	Lat.	3	$\frac{1}{4}$	3	$\frac{3}{4}$	3	2–3
	Through joint	Lat.	2	$\frac{1}{8}$	3	$\frac{1}{8}$	3	$\frac{1}{4}$
11	Femur	CrCd	2	$\frac{1}{8}$	2	$\frac{1}{4}$	3	$\frac{3}{8}$
		Lat.	1	$\frac{1}{8}$	3	$\frac{1}{8}$	3	$\frac{3}{8}$
	Through body	Lat.	1	$\frac{3}{16}$	3	$\frac{1}{4}$	3	$\frac{1}{2}$–$\frac{3}{4}$
12	Stifle	CrCd	1	$\frac{1}{8}$	2	$\frac{1}{8}$	3	$\frac{3}{16}$
		Lat.	1	$\frac{1}{8}$	1	$\frac{1}{8}$	2	$\frac{3}{16}$
	Trochlear gr.		1	$\frac{1}{8}$	1	$\frac{1}{8}$	2	$\frac{1}{8}$
13	Tibia and fibula	CrCd	1	$\frac{1}{8}$	1	$\frac{1}{8}$	2	$\frac{1}{4}$
		Lat.	1	$\frac{1}{8}$	1	$\frac{1}{8}$	2	$\frac{1}{4}$
14	Tarsus	DPl	1	$\frac{1}{8}$	2	$\frac{1}{8}$	3	$\frac{1}{4}$
		Lat.	1	$\frac{1}{8}$	1	$\frac{1}{8}$	2	$\frac{1}{4}$
15	Metatarsus	DPl	1	$\frac{1}{8}$	1	$\frac{1}{8}$	1	$\frac{1}{4}$
		Lat.	1	$\frac{1}{8}$	1	$\frac{1}{8}$	2	$\frac{1}{4}$
Skull								
16	General	VD	1	$\frac{1}{8}$	2	$\frac{1}{4}$	3	$\frac{1}{4}$
		DV	1	$\frac{1}{8}$	2	$\frac{1}{4}$	3	$\frac{1}{4}$
		Lat.	1	$\frac{1}{8}$	2	$\frac{1}{4}$	3	$\frac{1}{4}$
17	Cranium and sinuses	RCd	1	$\frac{1}{4}$	2	$\frac{3}{8}$	3	$\frac{1}{2}$
		VD	1	$\frac{1}{8}$	3	$\frac{1}{4}$	3	$\frac{1}{4}$–$\frac{5}{16}$

* Kodak Non-screen film.

A.E.I. (NEWTON-VICTOR) K.5 (G.E. F.4) 15 mA PORTABLE UNIT

Small animal

Standard screens.
Medium-speed film.
75 cm focal–film distance.
Apparatus operated at 15 mA.

Position No.	Part	View	5 kg		20 kg		40 kg	
			Stud	sec	Stud	sec	Stud	sec
19	Nasal chambers	VD	1	$\frac{1}{8}$*	1	$\frac{1}{8}$	2	$\frac{1}{8}$
20	Temporo-mandibular	Lat.	1	$\frac{1}{8}$	3	$\frac{3}{4}$	3	$\frac{1}{4}$
	joints	Obl.	1	$\frac{1}{8}$	3	$\frac{1}{8}$	3	$\frac{1}{4}$
	Teeth							
22	Upper incisors	IO*	1	$\frac{1}{4}$‡	2	$\frac{1}{4}$‡	3	$\frac{1}{4}$‡
	Upper molars	Obl.	1	$\frac{1}{8}$	3	$\frac{1}{8}$	3	$\frac{1}{4}$
	Upper molars	Open mouth	1	$\frac{1}{8}$	2	$\frac{1}{8}$	3	$\frac{1}{8}$
23	Lower incisors	IO*	1	$\frac{1}{4}$‡	2	$\frac{1}{4}$‡	3	$\frac{1}{4}$‡
	Lower molars	Open mouth	1	$\frac{1}{8}$	2	$\frac{1}{8}$	3	$\frac{1}{8}$
	Lower molars	Occ.†	1	$\frac{1}{8}$‡	1	$\frac{1}{8}$‡	1	$\frac{1}{4}$‡
Spine								
25	Cervical	VD	1	$\frac{1}{8}$	2	$\frac{3}{8}$	3	$\frac{1}{2}$
		Lat.	1	$\frac{1}{16}-\frac{1}{8}$	2	$\frac{1}{4}$	3	$\frac{3}{8}-\frac{1}{2}$
26	Cervico-thoracic	VD	1	$\frac{1}{8}$	3	$\frac{1}{4}$	3	$\frac{1}{2}$
		Lat.	1	$\frac{1}{8}$	2	$\frac{3}{16}$	3	$\frac{1}{2}-\frac{3}{4}$
27	Thoracic	VD	1	$\frac{1}{4}$	2	$\frac{3}{8}$	3	$\frac{1}{2}-\frac{3}{4}$
		Lat.	1	$\frac{1}{8}$	3	$\frac{1}{4}$	3	$\frac{1}{2}$
28	Thoraco-lumbar	VD	1	$\frac{1}{4}$	2	$\frac{3}{8}$	3	$\frac{1}{2}$
		Lat.	1	$\frac{1}{8}$	2	$\frac{1}{4}$	3	$\frac{1}{2}$
29	Sacrum	VD	2	$\frac{1}{4}$	3	$\frac{3}{4}$	3	$1\frac{1}{4}$
		Lat.	2	$\frac{1}{4}$	3	$\frac{1}{4}$	3	$\frac{1}{2}$
30	Coccyx	DV*	1	$\frac{3}{4}$	1	$\frac{3}{4}$	1	$\frac{3}{4}$
		Lat.*	1	$\frac{3}{4}$	1	$\frac{3}{4}$	1	$\frac{3}{4}$
Soft tissue								
2	Pharynx	Lat.	1	$\frac{1}{16}-\frac{1}{8}$	2	$\frac{1}{16}$	3	$\frac{1}{16}$
3	Lungs	DV	2	$\frac{1}{8}$	3	$\frac{1}{8}$	3	$\frac{3}{8}$
		Lat.	2	$\frac{1}{16}$	3	$\frac{1}{8}$	3	$\frac{1}{4}$
4	Abdomen	VD	3	$\frac{1}{4}$	3	$\frac{1}{2}$	3	$\frac{3}{4}-1$
		Lat.	2	$\frac{1}{8}-\frac{1}{4}$	2–3	$\frac{1}{4}$	3	$\frac{3}{8}-\frac{1}{2}$

* Kodak Non-screen film.
† Kodak Fast Occlusal film.
‡ 30 cm focal–film distance.

PHILIPS 'PRACTIX' 20 mA PORTABLE UNIT

Small animal

Standard screens.
Medium-speed film.
75 cm focal–film distance.
Apparatus operated at 20 mA.

Position No.	Part	View	5 kg		20 kg		40 kg	
			kV	sec	kV	sec	kV	sec
19	Nasal chambers	VD	55	0.16	65	0.25	70	0.25
20	Temporo-mandibular	Lat.	60	0.10	65	0.50	70	0.50
	joints	Obl.	60	0.10	65	0.50	70	0.50
	Teeth							
22	Upper incisors	IO*	50	0.16‡	60	0.16‡	60	0.20‡
	Upper molars	Obl.	60	0.10	65	0.25	70	0.30
	Upper molars	Open mouth	60	0.20	65	0.30	65	0.50
23	Lower incisors	IO*	50	0.16‡	60	0.16	60	0.20‡
	Lower molars	Open mouth	60	0.20	65	0.30	65	0.50
	Lower molars	Occ.†	50	0.40‡	60	0.40	60	0.60‡
Spine								
25	Cervical	VD	60	0.20	65	0.50	70	0.60
		Lat.	60	0.10	65	0.25	70	0.25
26	Cervico-thoracic	VD	65	0.20	75	0.50	85	1.00 Grid
		Lat.	60	0.10	70	0.30	80	0.80
27	Thoracic	VD	65	0.20	75	0.65	85	1.00 Grid
		Lat.	60	0.25	70	0.40	80	0.40
28	Thoraco-lumbar	VD	65	0.30	80	0.80	85	1.00 Grid
		Lat.	60	0.20	75	0.60	80	0.40
29	Sacrum	VD	60	0.20	65	0.50	70	0.50
		Lat.	60	0.20	70	0.25	80	0.40
30	Coccyx	DV	50	0.08	60	0.08	65	0.10
		Lat.	50	0.08	60	0.08	65	0.10
Soft tissue								
2	Pharynx	Lat.	55	0.08	70	0.10	80	0.10
3	Lungs	DV	80	0.08	80	0.16	90	0.16
		Lat.	70	0.04	80	0.08	80	0.10
4	Abdomen	VD	65	0.50	75	0.50	85	0.50
		Lat.	60	0.30	70	0.20	75	0.30

* Kodak Non-screen film.
† Kodak Fast Occlusal film.
‡ 30 cm focal–film distance.

PHILIPS 'PRACTIX' 20 mA PORTABLE UNIT

Average equine

Standard screens.
Medium-speed film.
75 cm focal–film distance.
8:1 grid used where indicated. Apparatus operated at 20 mA.

Position No.	Part	View	kV	sec
1	Distal phalanx	DPr-PaDi Obl.	60	0.08
2	Distal sesamoid	DPr-PaDi Obl.	75	1.20–1.60 Grid
3	Proximal and middle phalanges	DPa	70	0.20
		Lat.	70	0.20
4	Fetlock	DPa	75	0.30
		Lat.	70	0.25
	Proximal sesamoids	DPa	75	0.30
		Obl.	70	0.25
5	Metacarpus	Obl.	70	0.25
6	Carpus	DPa	70	0.30
	Extended	Lat.	70	0.25
	Flexed	Lat.	70	0.25
7	Tarsus	DPl	75	0.50
		Lat.	75	0.30
10	Elbow	CrCd	85	1.60
		Lat.	75	0.50
13	Shoulder	Obl.	90	1.60
		Lat.	90	1.00
14	Stifle	CdCr	90	2.00 Grid
		Lat.	65	0.60
16	Skull	VD	90	0.32
		R lat.	90	0.25
		Cd lat.	90	0.40
		Obl.	85	0.40
	Spine			
18	Cervical spine	Lat.	95	0.50
19	Thoracic processes	Lat.	75	0.25

S.M.R. 110/35 PORTABLE UNIT

Small animal

Standard screens.
Medium-speed film.
75 cm focal–film distance.

Position no.	Part	View	5 kg			20 kg			40 kg		
			kV	mA	sec	kV	mA	sec	kV	mA	sec
Forelimb											
1	Scapula	CdCr	75	20	0.12	90	15	0.16	90	15	0.2
		Lat.	60	25	0.08	75	20	0.16	90	15	0.1
2	Shoulder	Lat.	60	25	0.06	60	25	0.1	75	20	0.1
3	Humerus	CrCd	60	25	0.08	75	20	0.12	75	20	0.2
		CdCr	60	25	0.08	75	20	0.12	75	20	0.2
		Lat.	50	35	0.06	60	25	0.08	60	25	0.1
4	Elbow	CrCd	50	35	0.06	60	25	0.16	75	20	0.16
		Lat.	50	35	0.06	60	25	0.08	60	25	0.12
5	Radius and ulna	CrCd	50	35	0.06	60	25	0.08	60	25	0.1
		Lat.	50	35	0.06	50	35	0.08	60	25	0.1
6	Carpus	DPa	50	35	0.06	50	35	0.08	60	25	0.1
		Obl.	50	35	0.06	50	35	0.08	60	25	0.1
		Lat.	50	35	0.06	50	35	0.08	60	25	0.1
7	Metacarpus	DPa	50	35	0.06	50	35	0.08	60	25	0.1
		Lat.	50	35	0.06	50	35	0.08	60	25	0.1
8	Digits	DPa	50	35	0.06	50	35	0.08	60	25	0.1
		Lat.	50	35	0.06	50	35	0.06	50	35	0.1
Hindlimb											
10	Hip joint	VD	60	25	0.1	75	20	0.4	75	20	0.63
	Through pelvis	Lat.	60	25	0.16	75	20	0.4	75	20	0.63
	Through joint	Lat.	60	25	0.08	60	25	0.1	65	25	0.2
11	Femur	CrCd	60	25	0.1	60	25	0.1	75	20	0.3
		Lat.	50	35	0.08	60	25	0.1	65	25	0.16
	Through body	Lat.	60	25	0.16	75	20	0.1	75	20	0.63
12	Stifle	CrCd	60	25	0.08	60	25	0.1	75	20	0.16
		Lat.	50	35	0.06	60	25	0.08	60	25	0.12
	Trochlear gr.		50	35	0.04	50	35	0.06	60	25	0.08
13	Tibia and fibula	CrCd	50	35	0.06	60	25	0.1	60	25	0.16
		Lat.	50	35	0.06	60	25	0.08	60	25	0.12
14	Tarsus	DPl	50	35	0.06	60	25	0.1	60	25	0.12
		Lat.	50	35	0.06	60	25	0.08	60	25	0.12
15	Metatarsus	DPl	50	35	0.06	60	25	0.1	60	25	0.12
		Lat.	50	35	0.06	60	25	0.08	60	25	0.1
Skull											
16	General	DV	60	25	0.1	75	25	0.25	75	20	0.32
		VD	60	25	0.1	75	20	0.25	75	20	0.32
		Lat.	60	25	0.1	75	20	0.25	75	20	0.32
17	Cranium and sinuses	RCd	75	20	0.2	75	20	0.3	75	20	0.5
		VD	75	20	0.2	75	20	0.25	75	20	0.4
19	Nasal chambers	VD	50	35	0.1	75	20	0.2	75	20	0.2

S.M.R. 110/35 PORTABLE UNIT

Small animal

Standard screens.
Medium-speed film.
75 cm focal–film distance.

Position no.	Part	View	5 kg			20 kg			40 kg		
			kV	mA	sec	kV	mA	sec	kV	mA	sec
20	Temporo-mandibular joints	Lat.	60	25	0.1	75	20	0.25	75	20	0.4
		Obl.	60	25	0.1	75	20	0.25	75	20	0.4
	Teeth										
22	Upper incisors	IO*	50	35	0.1‡	60	25	0.16‡	60	25	0.16‡
	Upper molars	Obl.	60	25	0.1	75	20	0.2	75	20	0.25
	Upper molars	Open mouth	60	25	0.2	75	20	0.3	75	20	0.4
23	Lower incisors	IO*	50	35	0.1‡	60	25	0.16‡	60	25	0.16‡
	Lower molars	Open mouth	60	25	0.1	75	20	0.2	75	20	0.25
	Lower molars	Occ.†	50	35	0.3‡	60	25	0.4‡	60	25	0.6‡
Spine											
25	Cervical	VD	60	25	0.2	75	20	0.3	75	20	0.5
		Lat.	60	25	0.1	75	20	0.25	75	20	0.3
26	Cervico-thoracic	VD	60	25	0.2	75	20	0.3	90	15	1.0 Grid
		Lat.	60	25	0.2	75	20	0.2	75	20	0.4
27	Thoracic	VD	60	25	0.25	90	15	0.2	95	15	1.0 Grid
		Lat.	60	25	0.16	75	20	0.2	75	20	0.63
28	Thoraco-lumbar	VD	60	25	0.3	90	15	0.3	90	15	1.0 Grid
		Lat.	60	25	0.2	75	20	0.25	75	20	0.63
29	Sacrum	VD	60	25	0.2	75	20	0.4	75	20	0.63
		Lat.	60	25	0.25	75	20	0.3	75	20	0.63
30	Coccyx	DV	50	35	0.08	60	25	0.06	65	25	0.1
		Lat.	50	35	0.08	60	25	0.06	65	25	0.1
Soft tissue											
2	Pharynx	Lat.	50	35	0.1	75	20	0.08	75	20	0.1
3	Lungs	DV	75	20	0.06	110	10	0.04	110	10	0.08
		Lat.	75	20	0.04	90	15	0.04	90	15	0.1
4	Abdomen	VD	75	20	0.25	90	15	0.3	90	15	0.8 Grid
		Lat.	75	20	0.1	75	20	0.16	75	20	0.3

* Kodak Non-screen film.   *† Kodak Fast Occlusal film.*   *‡ 30 cm focal–film distance.*

S.M.R. 110/35 PORTABLE UNIT

Average equine

Standard screens.
Medium-speed film.
75 cm focal–film distance.
8:1 grid used where indicated.

Position No.	Part	View	kV	mA	sec
1	Distal phalanx	DPr-PaDi Obl.	60	25	0.1
2	Distal sesamoid	DPr-PaDi Obl.	75	20	1.2 Grid
		DPr-PaDi Obl.	75	20	1.6 Grid
3	Proximal and middle phalanges	DPa	75	20	0.2
		Lat.	75	20	0.16
4	Fetlock	DPa	75	20	0.32
		Lat.	75	20	0.2
	Proximal sesamoids	DPa	75	20	0.32
		Obl.	75	20	0.2
5	Metacarpus	Obl.	75	20	0.25
6	Carpus	DPa	75	20	0.25
	Extended and flexed	Lat.	75	20	0.25
		Obl.	75	20	0.25
7	Tarsus	DPl	75	20	0.5
		Lat.	75	20	0.32
10	Elbow	CrCd	75	20	0.6
		Lat.	75	20	0.25
13	Shoulder	Lat./obl.	90	15	2.0
14	Stifle	CdCr	90	15	2.5 Grid
		Lat.	75	20	0.6
16	Skull				
	Nasal chambers	VD	90	15	0.4
		Lat.	90	15	0.4
	Gutteral pouch area	Lat.	90	15	0.5
	Maxillary sinuses	Obl.	90	15	0.3
	Spine				
18	Cervical spine	Lat.	90	15	0.63
19	Thoracic processes	Lat.	75	15	0.32